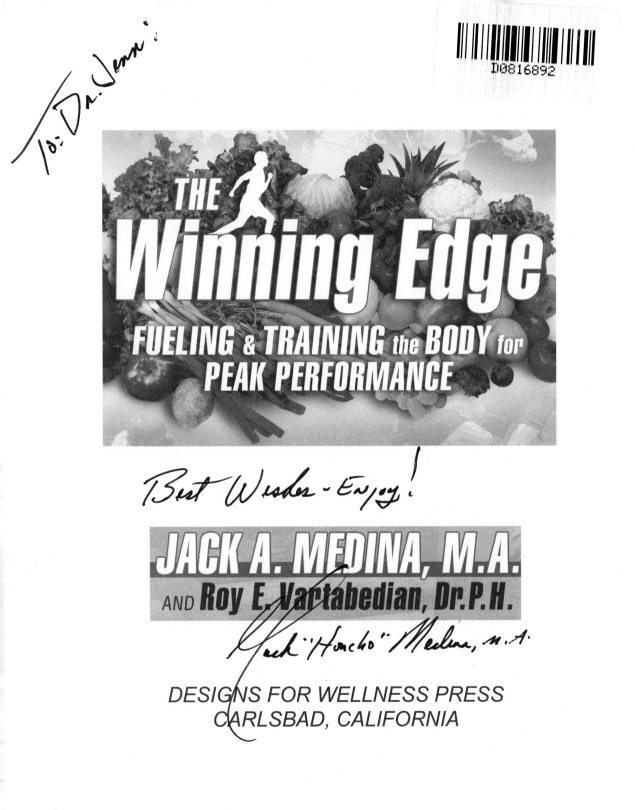

THE Winning Edge

FUELING & TRAINING the BODY for PEAK PERFORMANCE

To: Dr. Jenni

Best Wishes - Enjoy!

JACK A. MEDINA, M.A.
AND Roy E. Vartabedian, Dr.P.H.

Jack "Honcho" Medina, M.A.

DESIGNS FOR WELLNESS PRESS
CARLSBAD, CALIFORNIA

Second Edition, October, 2007

Copyright © 2002-2007

October, 2002, First Edition/First Printing
December, 2002, First Edition/Second Printing
March, 2003, First Edition/Third Printing
March, 2006, First Edition/Fourth Printing

By Jack A. Medina, M.A. and Dr. Roy E. Vartabedian
ISBN-13: 978-0-9641952-4-0

The information in this book reflects the authors' experience and current research. It is not intended to be used to replace or supercede individualized medical or professional advice. Before starting any nutrition or exercise program, you should consult a physician or other appropriate health professional to supervise your overall program.

Cover design by George Foster
FosterCovers.com

Printed in the United States of America

Other publications by the authors:

Nutripoints: Healthy Eating Made Simple!

More Fuel for the Winning Edge

PowerPack for the Winning Edge

Nutripoints & Optimal Nutrition

Visit our websites:
www.JackMedina.com
www.Nutripoints.com

DEDICATION

Why this book? Many years ago, when I was a young coach, there was a very famous gymnast in the United States named Cathy Rigby. Cathy was the first gymnast in the USA to ever win a medal in world class competition, Silver Medal on the Balance Beam at the World Championships. When Cathy retired from competition she started a gymnastics camp under her name at Wonder Valley Ranch in Sanger, California; California's first Dude Ranch. Cathy gave me the honor of asking me to be the Director of her camp and gave me the nickname "Honcho" since I was the head honcho at the camp. We had girls coming to us from all over the country, 125 per week, and they could stay for a week at a time up to 10 weeks.

We had one particular little girl (I will not use her name) come to camp. She was 10 years old, and her goal in life was to make the United States Olympic Team. We trained every day from 8:00 a.m. until noon and after lunch the kids could participate in one or more of the many activities available to them (swimming, water skiing, horseback riding, crafts, etc.). This little girl didn't want to do any of these activities, she wanted to workout. So I spent most of my time each afternoon working with her; she trained between 6 and 10 hours each day, virtually 7 days a week for 10 weeks every summer. At age 14, her 4th year in camp, she was good enough, in my opinion, to make the United States Olympic Team.

Some time later one of my fellow coaches, who worked with me at the camp, called to tell me the following: During the last week or so of this young girl's stay at camp her parents had moved from wherever it was they lived to an exclusive area in Southern California. They picked up their daughter on the last day of camp and drove down south. A day or so later they drove over to the local high school, dropped their daughter off and said, "Go tell them you're a new student," and drove away. What does this 14-year-old girl do? Where does she go? What happens after school? Does anyone pick her up, and if so at what time and where?

Under this stress she is found by some female students crying. Feeling sorry for her they strike up a conversation and finally ask, "What do you like to do for fun?" The young girl says, "I'm a gymnast and I'm going to make the United States Olympic Gymnastics Team this year." These girls looked her in the eye and said, "How can you make the Olympic Gymnastics Team when your legs are so fat?" She answered, "Honcho didn't say I was fat." They said, "We don't even know what a Honcho is. She answered, "That's my summer coach and he didn't say I was fat." "Well," one of the girls said, "obviously you're too fat, but we're too fat too and we have formed a new club here, not school sponsored, called the "Too Fat Club". All you have to do to join our club is take these diet pills with us. You'll get rid of your fat legs, we'll get rid of our fat, you can be in our club, and we'd love to have you."

The new girl thought, why would they lie to me, they just met me, I must be too fat. So, in order to be accepted into this new group, she started taking the diet pills. Well, her mother caught her with the pills and took them away; she got some more. Then she decided, if I stop eating while I'm taking these diet pills, I'll bet I can lose my fat legs faster, so she stopped eating. Her mother made her eat, so after the evening meal the girl would run into the bathroom, stick her thumb down her throat, and vomit the food up again.

I want you to read this carefully because it changed my life many years ago!

Three weeks from the day this young 14-year-old gymnast entered high school and began taking the diet pills to be accepted; three weeks from that day she was admitted into the local hospital in a severe state of anorexia or starvation. And three weeks later she **died!** The last words she said, before breathing her last breath was, "Get me Honcho!" She didn't ask for her parents, she didn't ask for her full-time coach, she didn't ask for a friend—she asked for me! I didn't even know she was sick! I didn't know anything about nutrition; in fact, if I had it in college I certainly don't remember it. They didn't even have exercise physiology when I went to college.

So, over this little 14-year-old's gravesite I made a promise to her that I would find out what happened inside her body. And I started to study nutrition and exercise physiology; I found out what happened and I have dedicated the rest of my life to that little girl.

I now travel worldwide speaking on "Fact and Fantasy in Nutrition and Exercise" hoping I can somehow prevent this kind of thing from happening again. That is why this book has been written!

Coach Medina (Honcho)

CONTENTS

FOREWARD

Jack Medina has been spanning the globe for 35-plus years preaching the gospel of personal fitness and health to hundreds of thousands of people. Known as "America's Personal Trainer", his motivating style has inspired countless lives to be changed for the better. He uses safe and effective methods for physical training, body fat loss, and nutritional improvement. Over the years, Jack has been asked a lot of questions about weight loss, body fat loss, training techniques, and supplements. People have asked how these and other methods have helped as he trained some of the world's finest gymnasts, including Olympic competitors.

In this book, *"The Winning Edge: Fueling & Training the Body for Peak Performance"*, Jack presents answers to many of these questions, providing up-to-date information for anyone interested in training safely and effectively to achieve optimal health. Even competitive athletes can benefit from Jack's insight and advice.

Dr. Roy Vartabedian has also lectured extensively worldwide for the past 25-plus years, working mainly in the area of education for optimal nutrition through better food choices. His groundbreaking "Nutripoints" program assigns a point value to foods, giving a quality score to every food and thus making it simple for people to make improved food choices. In this book, Dr. Vartabedian joins forces with Jack Medina using the Nutripoint method to evaluate and recommend the best foods for active individuals and athletes searching for optimal health and peak performance.

"The Winning Edge" is a valuable handbook not only for those with a physically active lifestyle but also for those just starting on the road to personal fitness and health improvement. These two speakers and authors have inspired me with their dynamic and knowledgeable presentations. As you read this book, I feel confident that you too, will be inspired to reach out and achieve your personal health and fitness goals! Best wishes!

Richard E. DuBois, MD, FACP, Chief, Internal Med., Atlanta Med. Ctr.

ACKNOWLEDGEMENTS

I would like to thank the following people who have contributed to this book and my life—Jack Medina

- My mother and father (Anna May & Ellsworth Conrad Medina), who are in heaven together. They gave me life, love, discipline and encouragement. They stood behind me when not many people did. I hope I made you proud!

- My wonderful wife Kathy for her love and support over the past 46 years. This book would not be possible without her encouragement.

- Our three children, now grown up. Marjorie, Kelly and Randy. They are such a very important part of my life. They have made me so proud to be their father. In addition, my five grandchildren: Nicole, Michelle, Michael, Brandi and Cassondra who make the future bright and fun.

- Coach Tony Schulmeyer my high school football coach at San Lorenzo Valley High School in Felton, California, 1955-1956. He set an example for me that I wanted to follow: to become a coach!

- The Fremont Union High School District, Sunnyvale, California. In 1962 they offered me my first teaching/coaching position at Homestead High School, Cupertino, California. I will be forever grateful!

- All of my coaches and teachers at San Jose State College who molded me as a man and had an impact on my life.

- Barry S. Brown, Ph.D., University of Arkansas—one of the finest Exercise Physiologists in the world and a personal friend. Early in my coaching career when I began to have serious questions about what I was teaching and coaching, Barry was there to help guide me. He is still doing it today!

- Every football player and gymnast I have ever coached over the past 38 years, and those I didn't coach but from whom I learned.

- The many people, too many to mention here, that have had or are still having an impact on my life. You know who you are! Thanks!

- Dr. Scott Connelly, M.D. - Stanford University Medical Center whom I met in the 1970's when I went to a nutrition seminar he was presenting. He opened my eyes to a new world of knowledge. He made nutrition easy to understand and me hungry to learn more. I took notes like crazy and much of this information, still valid today, is included in this book.

- Reverend Bob Richards - former Olympic Gold Medal Winner in the Decathlon, Sports Commentator and speaker. He had a tremendous influence on my life when I heard him speak in the mid 1960's on setting a goal, motivation and responding to challenges. Many of his thoughts, words and stories, as I remember them, are still true today and have become an important part of this book.

- Dr. Roy Vartabedian, Dr.P.H. - Co-author of this book and my personal friend. For his encouragement to take on this difficult task and for his continuing willingness to teach and guide me. Most importantly for honoring me with his friendship. This book was an impossibility without him.

- To you, the person reading this book. I sincerely hope the material within this manuscript will motivate you, encourage you and guide you to a longer, healthier lifestyle.

Jack Medina

ABOUT THE AUTHORS

Jack A. Medina, M.A.

Mr. Jack Medina is President of Designs for Fitness, a consulting firm dedicated to educating the public about nutrition, exercise, stress management and injury prevention. Jack Medina has been designing fitness programs for people of all ages and abilities for more than 35 years, lecturing throughout the world, inspiring thousands of people to take charge to improve their personal wellness and live more balanced healthy lives. His unique ability to motivate his audiences through his highly informative and entertaining seminars has brought him worldwide recognition and appreciation.

Jack Medina received his Bachelor's and Master's Degree in Physical Education from San Jose State University. He began his coaching career at Homestead High School in Cupertino, California. Moving on to California State University in Northridge, Jack developed 19 All-American gymnasts and 3 national event champions.

Later, he worked with many of the top gymnasts in the world, including the USA's Cathy Rigby. He also served as a strength and conditioning consultant for the Raiders, Rams, Seahawks and Warriors. Jack implemented and supervised a "Stress Management-Wellness" program for Los Alamos National Laboratory and their 10,000 employees.

Jack Medina is the author of numerous articles on health issues, an active member of the American College of Sports Medicine, the National Strength and Conditioning Association, and a Certified Fitness Specialist by the Cooper Aerobics Center in Dallas, Texas, one of the most prestigious in the world. Jack has worked with many of the best orthopedists, chiropractors and physical therapists in the world and has been the featured guest on many radio and television shows across the U.S., Canada, and Europe.

For More Information: www.JackMedina.com

Roy E. Vartabedian, Dr.P.H., M.P.H.

Dr. Roy Vartabedian is President of Vartabedian & Associates/ Designs for Wellness, a Health and Nutrition publishing and consulting firm. He is also a Doctor of Public Health, with a specialty in Chronic Disease Prevention from Loma Linda University, and holds Master of Public Health degrees in Health Education and Nutrition also from LLU. He has worked in the field of health promotion and disease prevention for over 25 years, working with patients, managing programs, consulting, and speaking throughout the U.S., Canada, Australia and New Zealand.

His landmark publication, **Nutripoints**, is a New York Times National Best-Seller, and has been used in a total of 13 countries in 10 languages worldwide. He has appeared on numerous T.V., and radio programs including the Today Show, Live with Regis, and Everyday with Joan Lunden. Articles on his Nutripoints Program have appeared in many publications including Ladies' Home Journal, New Woman, the New York Times, and the Dallas Morning News.

Previously, Dr. Vartabedian worked as Executive Director of Wellness Programs at the world-renowned Cooper Clinic in Dallas, Texas. There he worked with Dr. Kenneth Cooper to develop the residential lifestyle improvement program on the 30-acre Cooper Aerobics Center facility in Dallas, directing the program for 6 years.

Before working with Dr. Cooper, he taught Preventive Care in the Family Practice Residency at Florida Hospital, Orlando, Florida for 4 years. There he trained Family Practice physicians how to incorporate Patient Education and Preventive Medicine into their practices, and developed the award-winning Preventive Care Learning Center, a facility patients use to learn more about how to improve their health and understand their disease when visiting their doctor.

For More Information: www.Nutripoints.com

INTRODUCTION

There are over 250,000 supplements on the market today and 30+ new diets every month. Everyone is looking for some kind of edge, and are seemingly willing to pay any price for it—including risking their personal health. Ads and claims for various supplements and drugs are all over the television stations and "testimonial" ads for weight loss programs are everywhere.

Well, there is no easy way! Regardless of what you are told by manufacturers, very few supplements can actually make a difference in the performance capability of an athlete. The key is fueling and training the body properly. Training the correct energy systems to give the correct response is, in my opinion, critical.

It takes dedication and hard work to be successful in any endeavor, in this case fueling and training the body for success—there is no "pill" for success.

Knowing what works and doesn't work is important and that is why this book has been written.

After the first 7 years of my own coaching career, which started in 1962, I thought I was pretty knowledgeable. After meeting Dr. Barry Brown, Ph.D. (Exercise Physiology) at the University of Arkansas at a conference, I found out I knew very little about what actually happens inside the body during exercise, which energy system did what and how to train it. What does three sets of 10 repetitions really mean in weight training, what is the difference between strength, power, muscular endurance, quickness and speed?

I didn't understand how important fueling the body is to reaching peak performance, what a carbohydrate is, what it did and why it did it. Then I had the opportunity to meet Dr. Roy Vartabedian, Dr.P.H., M.P.H., formerly responsible for the nutrition program at the famous Cooper Aerobic Center in Dallas, Texas and author of the Nutripoints Program for Optimal Nutrition. I quickly found out how much I didn't know and how easy it could be to fuel the body so it can function maximally.

Now, when I do "Fueling and Training The Body For Peak Performance" seminars throughout the U.S. and worldwide, hoping to share what I've learned over 45+ years, it's amazing how many coaches are not in attendance. Maybe they aren't as hungry to learn as I was or just don't want to give up the time.

So, with the help, encouragement, and partnership of Dr. Roy Vartabedian, the idea of writing this book came about. Since the first printing, new ideas and important information have become available. This book has been written to share with you, so you and the athlete can reach peak performance.

CHAPTER ONE

ON TO VICTORY

Do you have a goal relative to your health, nutrition and exercise, or sports performance? I would like to share with you the quest for life's higher goals, believing that out of the sports world, the world of muscle and bone, grit and grime, you can see life written large as boys and girls, men and women struggle for goals, hurting, in pain, but going "On to Victory". I think that what happens on an athletic field or in a gymnasium or on a court is exactly what happens in living. What takes place on a ball diamond or track; these are the struggles in life. Everyone wants to be a champion in one endeavor or another. Everyone's playing the great game—the game of life, and I believe the sports world can speak to each and every one of us. Also, I believe the sports world can speak to our culture.

I may be stretching the sports category, but I believe we live in a world of mediocrity, when people are prone to throw things together in a slip-shod way. I love the sports world because you can't be successful by being mediocre. You've got to go beyond the ordinary, you've got to reach out and try to excel. I love the sports world because in our world of the passive you've got to get active. We live in a time when people try to let life mold them. A full-page ad illustrated this for me not long ago: "Now you don't have to exercise yourself, you just lay on this machine and it exercises you!" Sound familiar?

Well, in the sports world you've got to get active. You have to take life, so to speak, by the horns. You have to get out there and run, you've got to do push-ups, chin-ups and lift weights. You can't sit around and daydream in the locker-room; you can't sit in the stands and criticize. Pretty soon you have to go out there and hurt and take the action in your own hands. In the sports world you have to put your ideas into muscle, you've got to act upon what you know.

We live in a time when people tend to forget the individual in giant corporations and institutions. But in the sports world, football for example, the guard can't rely on the tackle to do his job for him. The quarterback can't rely on the fullback. Each and every player must do their assigned task and the team only functions when every individual does what he or she is supposed to do. You see, underneath the team there is a person, an individual functioning. This is a great lesson, that underneath society there are individuals and you only change society when individuals live up to their responsibilities.

I love the sports world, because in an age of something for nothing, it says you only get out of it what you put into it. People are prone to think that circumstances in life will change their fortune. Well, in the sports world you only get out of it what you put into it, the number of hours spent running; you can only run as long as those lungs are trained to go, you can only jump as high as those muscles will lift you. In other words you must rely on work, discipline, and faith. You can't rely on something for nothing.

It is also a world of struggle, and I don't personally believe that a boy or girl, man or woman is prepared for life until they are prepared for knocks and bumps and bruises. Life is not easy. The person who will succeed in life must learn this: you've got to hurt! You've got to go through the sweat, blood and tears so to speak. The sports world can teach you this. You are prepared to face obstacles. Anyone who has run a race and gone out for a record knows what it is like when those lungs are pounding and there is lactic acid in your muscles and you're tired. Well, that's life!

You only understand life if you see it as a struggle, the struggle for life's higher goals. Believing that out of the sports world you can see life emerge, you can see life written large. So the first thing I want to say here is this: If you want to accomplish much in sport or any realm of life you've got to get a goal, a high one, you've got to keep your eyes on that goal, and you've got to follow through with all you've got. Now this is simple isn't it?

Any of you who have participated in sports know the axiom of the sports world—keep your eyes on the ball, follow through. The great golfers in history will tell you they work on two things: they pinpoint the back of that ball, meet it with the club firmly, and the six inches in front of the ball, follow through straight towards that pin. Any phenomenon in sport can be summarized by these words: keep your eye on the goal—follow through!

A goal can pull out every ability you have. It makes every step meaningful, every chin-up, every push-up, every bit of weight training; it gives it purpose. You've got to have a goal! You've got to have something to pull you out regardless of how tremendous it is. Dreams can come true!

Now of course the hard part is the follow-through. I don't know if you are aware of this or not, but in Scandinavia whenever a runner runs, the whole crowd runs with him. They vicariously identify with the runners. One of the world's greatest track athletes from Scandinavia was Emil Zatopek who would literally run with the crowd; 70,000 of them, all stomping their feet in unison, clapping their hands, yelling Zat-O-Pek, Zat-O-Pek, Zat-O-Pek! And you could watch this guy down on the track as he keeps pace with the people in the stands. Half way through the race the people speed up the chant and the guy is sweating but picks up the pace and holds the chant with the people. The last lap or so the entire stands are screaming Zatopek, Zatopek, Zatopek and here is this guy, tired, worn-out, a mask of torture, driving down to the finish-line! They have driven him to world's records.

Picture this! A guy is involved in a half-mile race, the finals of the 800 meters. Eight guys are coming out of the starting blocks, all of them wide eyed with excitement as each boy has worked his way through the qualifying heats, quarterfinals, semi-finals and now the race for the Gold Medal. Five of these guys are World Record Holders. You talk about tension! Arnie Soul from Villanova sets a terrific pace as he takes the lead into the curve. Down the backstretch and into the next curve Arnie gives everything he has to keep the pace going and that's his mistake; and you can only make one in the Olympic Games. Behind him is the World Record Holder from Norway. Just behind him the great runner from Great Britain, and just behind him Lonnie Spurrier from California. Five World Record Holders begin giving everything they've got.

As they come into the final curve they hit the "wall"; the pace was too fast! With 110 yards left to go four guys catch Arnie Soul and as they finish the curve a terrific gust of wind blows down the track and almost stops them in their tracks. Tom Courtney said, "Just as I finished the curve and entered the straightaway I ran completely out of gas."

You coaches and athletes know what this is. The sickening feeling of fatigue when your lungs are burning and your mouth is dry, as you feel numb all over. You want to go on, you can see the finish line; the spirit, while it is very willing, the flesh is so weak. Tom Courtney said he just hoped everyone else was just as tired as he was when all of a sudden Johnson from Great Britain forged around him and went out in front by two yards.

The question is what happens to a guy in a moment like that? It's easy to let down in the fatigue, easy to say, "I'll settle for second." What happens to a guy when he says, as Tom Courtney said, "I had to win that race! My goal was to win this race." This guy, muscles filled with lactic acid, almost all of the oxygen gone out of his blood, but running out of the heart, the emotional desire.

This guy picked his knees up, fought his way back and caught Johnson with 10 yards left to go. I wish you could see a slow motion shot of just one picture, the picture of a guy coming into the tape almost unconscious, his eyes closed, teeth set, every muscle rippling; the guy drives towards the tape, lunges out, hits it and collapses, beating Johnson by 6 inches in the deafening roar of the crowd. He could hardly walk off the track after the race; they had to postpone the victory ceremony for an hour.

If you want to hear about desire and heart, how about a basketball player named Willis Reed of the New York Knicks. The story goes like this: "And then Reed fell. Driving for the basket with only 8 minutes played, with no one near him, in the fifth game of the 1969-70 NBA playoff finals, he suddenly collapsed and lay still." Reed's face was twisted in pain and 19,500 people held their collective breath, including a nationwide television audience (I was in that audience). Every Knick fan could see their championship lying on the floor. Reed tried to stand, and pain ripped through his thigh. He had to leave the game and didn't return. Somehow the Knicks miraculously won the game and now there were two days left before the sixth game and seventh game and the Knicks held a 3 - 2 series lead.

Could Reed, the league's "Most Valuable Player", and the team's leading scorer, recover for either of those games? Reed couldn't play in game six because he could barely walk and was in so much pain; he didn't even suit up. Their opponent, the Lakers, defeated the Knicks easily in game six, tying the series with one game remaining. No one, including Willis Reed himself knew if he would play in the Championship game until he tried to test his leg during the warm-up, after which his comment was, "It hurts." He received a shot of cortisone and a pain killer in the locker room from the trainer and literally dragged his right leg behind him as he came back on the court for the start of the game. He was thinking, "I have to play a man six inches taller than me, stronger than me, a man who just had a 45-point game. I can't run and I can't jump, and somehow I'm supposed to compensate for all that."

He took a pass after the opening tip-off and scored the game's first basket, a 22-foot one-hander. The crowd was on its feet and screaming. Reed took another pass with only 83 seconds gone and popped in a second one-hander. He had taken two shots and scored both times. The Knicks now led 5-2 and the Lakers were finished. Reed somehow kept the great Wilt Chamberlain away from the basket, playing on nerve and pride. The rest of the Knicks darted superbly around Reed literally stunning the Lakers. Reed remained on the floor for about 20 minutes with an injury that defied painkillers. He just limped around the floor dragging his right leg.

Reed, who was interviewed by Frank Gifford for television right after the game said, "I was going to go out there and play. All of my life was that one game. Waiting for me was the greatest center who ever played the game. I had an obligation to myself and I had a responsibility, I had to help. The pain was still there. It never left me. I couldn't run, I couldn't jump or shoot, but I had to be there. People talk of choice. I had no choice." WOW!

What does Willis Reed want to be remembered for today? The answer came quickly. "There were a lot of things I couldn't do to my personal satisfaction in basketball, but what I could do, I did 100 percent. That's the only thing I'd like people to remember about me." What he could do, he did."

What's in a story like this? More than just physiology going through the motions. Here you see the basis for every great endeavor in life, the desire that drives a man or woman on through the hurt and pain to Victory! Out of a race like that comes a drama about what each and every person must have if they are going to accomplish anything in living. A burning desire must grip you to achieve a goal. You have to have the kind of will, the kind of heart that can respond.

You can't just go through the motions; you've got to follow-through with all you've got. Forgive this personal reference but in over 30 years of teaching and coaching I've spent more than 10,000 hours studying and learning. Men—women, you want to be something in life? You want to be a scholar, great in the sports world, you want to be a doctor, a lawyer, anything in life; you want to be great in business, put 10,000 hours of work into it and see what happens to your life. Here is one of the great axioms of sports, get a goal, keep your eyes on that goal and you must follow through with work, with all you've got.

But the sports world says you will be frustrated. I know this is a hard one. We like to talk about the champions, the person who wins the Gold Medal, the winning team—but the sports world is bigger than newspaper clippings. It talks about frustration, it talks about guys and girls giving everything they've got and they still lose by an inch or a point. It talks about athletes running down to the nub and they still fail. There are frustrating moments like this in life.

I think of a guy named Jim Peters running the race of his life, 20 minutes ahead of everyone else, he broke into the stadium in Vancouver, Canada. He had run 26 miles, the Marathon, on his way to a World's Record. But in 95-degree heat, lactic acid in his muscles, just as he made the turn into the roar of the crowd, 385 yards to go, he collapsed. He struggled to his feet, tried to go on but couldn't. Sixteen times fell down; when he couldn't get up anymore this guy crawled on his hands and knees to a white line he thought was the finish- line, and collapsed over it, 200 yards short of his goal.

Now you can't go up to a kid like that and say, "You've got to put out a little bit more," you just can't do it. There are times when a person puts out everything they have and still fail, they still don't win. But in the striving, in the development of a will that goes down that deep, a man or woman learns a great lesson about life. That somehow there can be more victory in a striving like that than there is in victory itself. And even beyond that I will predict that there can be defeat in victory if a person doesn't learn this.

This may sound strange but let me illustrate. Which one of these fellows would you rather be? A 6 foot 4 inch guy that weighed 195 pounds, could high jump 6' 8", long jump 25 feet, run the hundred meters in 10.2 seconds; he was enormous, he could do anything—big, fast. Would you rather be a boy like that who experts claimed would break every record, or a kid with a cut foot, cut so badly that every time he ran a race it hurt him, which one of those would you rather be?

Which one of these: An All-American his junior year at the University of Illinois, broke every one of Red Grange's football records, or would you rather be a kid 132 pounds, denied a uniform because he was too small and had a clubfoot, which one of those?

Which one of these? An Olympic Champion with a Gold Medal around his neck, waving at 110,000 people in victory, or would you rather be a boy that was supposed to win, wound up fourth and they lowered the British flag to half- mast?

Before you make up your mind let me tell you about these 6 boys.

The guy with all the ability in the world never made the Olympic Team, lost his temper repeatedly, walked off the track, wouldn't even finish his race; fighting coaches, officials, everyone. The other boy was Rafaer Johnson who went on to a World Record and Gold Medal in the Decathlon, in spite of that cut foot. He is still recognized today as one of the greatest athletes of all time.

The All-American halfback didn't even finish school. He took himself so seriously, he thought he couldn't play with his buddies, dropped out of school and they haven't seen him since. The other boy at 132 pounds, the kid with the clubfoot, Jack Hackett, went on to make All-State Pennsylvania, 2nd Team All-American and spent many years coaching at the University of Florida, molding men.

The guy with the Olympic Gold Medal committed suicide 6 months later, Cornelius Johnson, the 1936 High Jump Champion. The other boy was Roger Bannister who the following year became the first man in history to run the mile under 4 minutes!

You can't tell me that there can't be victory in defeat and that there can't be defeat in victory depending on the attitude you have. It isn't where you are going that counts, it's the direction in which you are headed! One of the great things about the sports world is that it can teach you to take frustration and come back out of it and go on to Victory. It's a great lesson to learn about life!

Lastly, you've got to hang on. You will be frustrated, but you must stay in there and battle. The sports world is filled with so many beautiful stories of it. I think of two football players during my early years: one of them Andy Robestelli and the other Johnny Unitas. Andy Robestelli, dropped by the Los Angeles Rams, was told he wasn't good enough; decided he was going to work harder than ever before. Seven consecutive years he made All Pro Defensive End with the New York Giants.

Johnny Unitas was turned down by several colleges, and wound up at the University of Louisville. He was a 5th round draft choice by the Pittsburgh Steelers; their 5th string Quarterback, and then dropped from the team, they didn't want him. All along, he kept in shape when virtually no one knew he even existed. Coach Weeb Eubank, who was building a championship team with the Baltimore Colts, wrote in a newspaper, "We're going to build a championship team if we can find a Quarterback." On a postcard, Johnny Unitas wrote, "Give me a chance coach; I know I can do it if you will just give me a chance." There was a telephone call back and Johnny Unitas was signed. Two years later he was named the Outstanding Football Player in the World!

That's what I mean by hanging on. You've got to stay in there and battle. If you get beneath the statistics of Victory and Defeat you will discover this: It's the hanging on that does it! There can be victory in defeat if you will just stay in there and battle and keep pressing on towards your goal.

Lastly, go for more than world records, more than profits in business or more than just learning in education, although these are all good in the right perspective. But I'm talking about something infinitely greater. Reach out for the highest goals there are—God, Character, and Morality! There is a spiritual something that throbs through many of our great athletes. They are what they are because of what they are in spirit. Bud Wilkinson, the former great football coach at the University of Oklahoma put it this way: "You show me a boy with a Spiritual Commitment and I'll show you a better football player. The discipline of his life will be greater, he'll work harder." Somehow when a divine dimension touches your life, it makes a difference.

MY PERSONAL MOTIVATION

My idol when I was in high school, college and when I began my coaching career in 1962 was the great Hall of Fame Coach Vince Lombardi of the Green Bay Packers. He is, in my mind, still in that same position today.

Coach Lombardi made a "Farewell" speech, on February 26, 1969, in Janesville, Wisconsin that touched me deeply. I want to paraphrase his message and share it with you. What he said then, still applies to you and me today!

"I have been in football all of my life, really, and I do not know whether I'm particularly qualified to do anything else, except to be a part of what I consider a great game. It is a great game, and I think it is a game of leaders, and I think it is a game which is a symbol of what is country's best attributes are, and that is courage, stamina, and coordinated efficiency.

And besides, it is a Spartan game. What I mean by that is it takes Spartan-like qualities in order to play it. The Spartan quality of sacrifice, and the Spartan quality of self-denial in particular. And it is a game of violent contact, yet because of that violent contact it demands a personal discipline, which is seldom found in any other place in this modern world. It is more than the National Football league, it is the people who grow up to make that league, it is the Hustons, and the Thorpes, and the Starrs, and the Giffords, and the hundreds of more like them. And it is the thousands upon thousands of high school and college players who take part in it annually. And it is the millions more, like you and I, who watch it from the sidelines or on TV.

And regardless of what level it is played upon, it exemplifies those attributes I mentioned...in addition to that, it has the means and the power to provide a physical and mental relaxation to those of us who watch it.

It was my good fortune, when I was at West Point for so many years, to get to know General Douglas MacArthur. Each Monday evening I would be asked by Coach Red Blaik to take the film of Saturday's game down to the Waldorf Towers, to show the General. He said many things to me about competitive sports, football in particular. He said it keeps alive a spirit of vitality, and enterprise. He was talking about everybody who was interested in the game. He said it teaches the strong to know when they are weak, and the brave to face themselves when they are afraid, to be proud, and to be unbending in defeat, yet humble and gentle in victory, and to master ourselves before we attempt to master others, to learn to laugh yet never forget how to weep, and it gives a predominance of courage over timidity.

I think those were great words from a great American, and there are other lessons, too. For example, I do not know of another game which in its early season requires the exhaustive hard work, to the point of drudgery, really, that the game of football requires. It is a game of team action, where the only reward that an individual gets is the total satisfaction that he is a part of the successful whole.

It is a game which gives 100-percent elation, it is a game which gives 100-percent fun, it is a game which is 100-percent laughter when you win, and yet extracts, and demands, really, a 100-percent resolution, a 100-percent determination, when you lose. It is a game of quick decisions; it is a game of strategy. It is a game that requires each man that is part of it to give something to the spirit of the team, because it is this very spirit that takes 11 hardened and talented men and binds them into a cohesive force. In this, I think is a great deal like life, in that it demands that a man's personal commitment must be to excellence, and must be to victory, even though you know that ultimate victory can never be completely won, yet that victory must be wooed, and it must be pursued with all of one's might.

And each week is a new encounter, each year there is a new challenge, yet all of the running, all of the color, and all of the glamour, and all of the excitement, these things linger only in the memory, but the spirit, the will to excel, the will to win, these are the things that endure.

Indeed I think that a quality of life is this full measure of a man's personal commitment to excellence and to victory, whether it be to football, whether it be in business, or whether it be in government, and I think there is a great need in this country for this kind of quality leadership in business, in politics, and in government.

And I think, too, it is like life; it teaches that work, and sacrifice, and perseverance, and competitive drive, and selflessness, and a respect for authority is the price that each and every one of us must pay to achieve any goal that is worthwhile.

A man must decide, and when I speak about man, I speak about you and me. A man must decide whether we want to provide a full life for humanity or destroy ourselves with our own problems.

And I think we must preserve what has always been an American zeal, and that is to be first, regardless of what we do, and to win, and to win, and to win.

You know, we speak about freedom, all of us do, we see it in the papers. All over the campuses it is freedom of speech, and freedom of this, it is the right to dissent, and all of these things, but I am afraid that sometimes, in my opinion, we confuse freedom with license. I think before any one of us can embrace freedom, we must first embrace those things which underline freedom, and I'm speaking about duty, I am speaking of respect for authority, and I am speaking of a development of a strong mental discipline.

These are the things that must first be embraced before we can embrace freedom.

And I am sure that you, like me, at times must be completely shocked by what seems to be a complete breakdown of law and order, and of moral code. It is almost beyond belief, and it is an unhappy thought, that our youth, the most gifted segment of our population, the inheritors of all our scientific advances and freedoms, the beneficiaries of all their elders' sacrifices and achievements, this small segment of youth—seems to have complete disregard for the indispensability of law and authority to their enjoyment and fullness of life.

And then they are joined with a certain group of their elders, who we think should know better, to seek a new right. I am still puzzled as to what that right is, but it seems to be a right to violate the laws of impunity, and the prevailing sentiment seems to be if you do not like the rule, break it.

I think it could be that the people who would lead us no longer understand the difference between themselves and the people, that while most shout to be independent, at the same time they wish to be dependent. And where most shout to assert themselves, at the same time they wish to be told what to do.

I want to talk about this phase of it, about the leadership phase of it, the quality of leadership. And when we speak of leadership, we are speaking about a position of command, and the doctrine of command can be summed up in one word—*leadership*, and leadership is defined as the ability to direct people, but more important to have that direction accepted. I think you and I both know that this is much too simple a definition for what is a very complex subject. I think most of us possess leadership ability, but unfortunately, leadership rests not on ability and not upon capacity; having ability and capacity are not enough; leadership is based on a willingness to use it.

And if it is said, it is then based upon truth, and upon character, and there must be truth in its purpose, and willpower in its character. Leadership rests not only upon ability, and not only upon capacity, but it also rests upon commitments, it rests upon loyalty, it rests upon pride, and it rests upon followers. We need leaders who will meet problems, intricate problems, with wisdom and with courage. Leaders, contrary to the opinion of many, are not born, they are made, and they are made just like everything else is made—by an effort and a price that we all pay to achieve any goal.

But at the same time the talented are no more responsible for their birthright than the underprivileged are, but the measure of each should be what each does in a specific situation.

And I want to say that has become increasingly difficult, to be tolerant of a society which seems to have sympathy only, and I emphasize that word, seems to have sympathy for only the misfit, for the maladjusted, for the criminal, and for the loser. Help them, have sympathy for them, yes, but I think it is also time to stand up and to cheer for, and to pat on the back those who recognize problems and do something about them, one who looks for something extra to do for his country.

I think above everything else, a man who would lead must be honest with himself, he must realize that he is just like everyone else, he must identify himself with the group, and he must back up that group even at the risk of displeasing some of his superiors. He must believe that the group wants from him a sense of approval, and I think if this prevails, you will find that production, and discipline, and morale will be high.

In return, you can demand the cooperation to promote the goals of your team, of your school, of your country, of your business, etc. You've got to believe in teamwork through participation.

You have to be sensitive to the emotional needs of others, and in return the attitude toward the leader will be one of confidence.

But in spite of what I've said, the leader can never really close the gap between himself and the people he leads.

And the most important element in the character makeup of a leader, and one of the most difficult to explain, is one of mental toughness, which is many things. Mental toughness is humility. It has qualities of sacrifice and self denial, and dedication, and fearlessness, and love. I'm not speaking here of a love that a man has for his wife, or wife for a husband, the love I'm speaking of is loyalty, which is the greatest of love. The love I speak of is teamwork; the love I speak of is the respect that one man has for the dignity of another man.

You show me a man who belittles another, and I'll show you a man who will never lead. You show me a man who is not charitable, and I will show you a man who will never lead.

And when all is said and done, I think a leader must exercise an effective influence upon the people that he leads, and the degree he accomplishes this depends upon the personality of the man.

But no leader, regardless of how great he may be, can long continue to lead unless he wins battles, because the battle decides all. Battles are won in the hearts of men, they will follow you anywhere.

The new leadership is in sacrifice, it is in self-denial, it is in love, it is in loyalty, it is in fearlessness, in humility, it is in the perfectly defined will.

This is not only the new leadership, this is the distinction between great and little men.

THANK YOU."

****

I close with this one last story. Coach Lou Little tells it about his greatest football team at the University of Columbia. They were on their way to the Conference Championship, just one last game. They had a boy on the squad who couldn't make the first team for four straight years. Just before the game, three days before, Lou was given a telegram to give to this boy saying that his only living relative had just died. The boy looked at the telegram and said, "Coach, I'll be back for Saturday's game."

The morning of the game the boy came up to Lou and said, "I want you to put me into this game, I know I haven't made the first team yet, but let me in for the kick-off and I'll prove to you I'm worthy of it." Well, Lou could see that the boy was disturbed and he made all kinds of excuses, but finally thought, "He can't do any harm on the kick-off." So he put the boy in.

The crowd roared as Columbia kicked off. The opposing halfback took the ball on the goal line; on the 7-yard line there was a tremendous tackle! The boy had dropped him in his tracks. Lou left him in. He made the next tackle, the next tackle, and the next tackle. He was all over the field; you couldn't move him out of there. He was an All-American that day and was the reason Columbia won the championship.

When the game was over and the celebration ended, only two people were left in the locker-room, coach Lou Little and this young boy. Coach Little walked over to this boy, put his arm around his shoulders and said, "I don't understand it, you haven't done anything for four straight years and today you're an All-American, what happened?" This young boy looked up at his coach with tears in his eyes and said, "Coach, you knew my Dad died didn't you?" Coach Little said, "Yes, I brought you the telegram." The boy said, "Well you knew my Dad was blind, didn't you?" Lou said, "Yes, I've seen you walk him around the campus many times." The boy said, "Coach, today's the first football game my Father ever saw me play!"

It makes a difference when those unseen eyes are watching!

There is Victory for you in terms of making your body healthy. It takes good nutrition and proper training but you can do it. So go on to victory by turning the pages, absorb the material and enjoy!

TRAINING/NUTRITION MYTHS & FACTS

How many people do you know that have ever been on a DIET? How many do you know that are no longer on that diet? How many do you know that started a diet, quit and are fatter now than they were when they started? Have you ever looked at the first 3 letters of that word? DIE! When you go on a diet with the expressed intent to lose weight, your body doesn't know you are going on a diet. Your body thinks you are trying to kill it and will do everything in its power to stop you from doing it.

In Search of the Magic Pill

If I had only one recommendation to make to you it would be "Don't Diet" just to lose weight, because when you do this your body thinks you are trying to commit suicide. If there was a "fat-loss pill" or "fat burning pill" that actually did what the advertising said, with no adverse side effects, maintained lean body tissue and was supported with good scientific research that was published in professional journals and presented to professional groups, don't you think this would be headline news all over the world?

If there really was one of these that worked, it would appear in the New England Journal, the American College of Sports Medicine, the National Strength and Conditioning Association, and many other professional journals. Why are there over 250,000 supplements available today, being advertised on television, radio, internet, and magazines? Simply because people are looking for a MAGIC pill; an easy way! Well there is no easy way! There are only gullible people who are easily swayed by the advertising being done, looking for an effortless way. These people want to be able to lay on it, sit on it, shake in it, vibrate in it, get wrapped up in it, or ingest it to get in shape. Well, you can't do it that way! It takes a common sense approach between eating good foods and exercise.

The Four Question Test

I want to give you something to take with you. I want to give you "**Four Questions**". So the next time you are in the mall and see a new diet product being advertised, or see a sign on a telephone pole saying "Lose up to 30 Pounds in 30 Days for 30 Dollars" or "We'll Pay You to Lose Weight", or "I Lost 42 Pounds in Two Weeks", etc., ask the following four questions. If whomever you are talking to can answer all four of these correctly, keep listening! If they miss one, I suggest you get away as fast as you can.

Number One: <u>How many calories does it take coming into MY body every day, via the food system, to keep me alive?</u>

If someone gives you a number, walk away. This is not correct. If you want to figure out how much energy you need, take your best weight (the weight you would be at if you could weigh anything you wanted to, instantly) and add a zero to that number. This gives you a close estimate of your BMR (Basal Metabolic Rate).

In other words the number of calories necessary coming into your body via the food system to keep you living at this body weight assuming you are laying in bed 24 hours a day doing absolutely nothing; just to keep your heart, brain, liver, kidneys, etc., doing what they are supposed to be doing.

Isn't it interesting that the average diet being promoted on radio and television, in newspapers and magazines and, on telephone poles in this country and many others is between 800 and 1000 calories or less? I will guarantee you that if I put you on 800 calories you WILL LOSE WEIGHT. You have to because you have less energy coming in than it takes to keep you alive. The question is: "For How Long Will I Lose This Weight?" Sooner or later you reach a "dietary plateau!" You are no longer losing, in fact you are gaining again because your body thinks it is dying and tries to save itself by turning everything that comes in to FAT and stores it.

The **Second question** is: <u>How Many Pounds of Fat Can I Lose on Your Program in 7 Days?</u>

The maximum amount of FAT the Human Body can lose in 7 days, regardless of what you are told is 3.3 pounds or a MIRACLE; without a MIRACLE 1 or 2 pounds is very good. But, someone you know goes on some new diet; and if you are looking for a new one, they average about 30 new ones each month, just look in the tabloids.

By the way, there is another new diet coming out that you may have an interest in. It is going to be called the "Combination Diet". What they have done is taken every known diet there is and put them all together in a giant mixer and finally into one can. It's going to be called, are you ready for this? "The XYZ-Supersaver-National Special-Lose It While You Sleep-Grapefruit Diet, manufactured by Lay On It, Sit On It, Shake In It, Vibrate In It, Get Wrapped Up In It, Rub It On Your Body, or Ingest It and Get In Shape Company!" It's a "BIG" can because the label information goes around 3 times!

The advertising goes like this: "Lose A Pound A Day"...this is not false advertising because I can put you on a diet and you can lose a pound a day, sometimes up to 30 or 40 days; but you CANNOT lose a pound of "FAT" per day. This is physiologically not possible! The advertising left out a very important word, "FAT".

Someone you know goes on this diet, and we will pick 7 days just for fun. In 7 days this person loses 7 pounds. At the end of the 7th day you notice some physical changes in this person as their face begins to "fall off"; their skin doesn't fit; they are grumpy and irritable, but they are LIGHTER—which is what they wanted in the first place!

Anyway, in 7 days they lose 7 pounds. Of the 7 pounds they lost, we will give them 2 pounds of fat, that's possible. They are going to lose a pound of water no matter what. But they lost 4 pounds of <u>something</u>. Everyone says they lost 4 pounds of MUSCLE! Not true! They didn't lose 4 pounds of muscle; they lost 4 pounds of PROTEIN.

Unfortunately every cell in your body is made up of some form of protein; which means this person's body ate itself inside out 4 pounds worth. They try to stay at this new weight as long as possible and it lasts about 3 weeks. Starving to death, skin not fitting, grumpy and irritable they say the heck with it, "I quit" and they do what 98% of people do who go on so-called quick diets, they go back to what they were eating in the first place.

The first thing their body puts back on after they quit the diet and start re-feeding is either the protein, water or fat. What do you think it is? FAT? No! WATER? No! Your body puts the PROTEIN back first. Why? Because every cell in your body is composed of some form of protein; there is no cellular growth without it, not any, and your body knows it—so it puts the PROTEIN back first. But with the 4 pounds of protein comes the one pound of WATER and the 2 pounds of FAT.

So now you are just as fat as you were when you started. Not this person. This person ends up 16 pounds fatter. How? Because it takes up to 4 pounds of water to re-metabolize one pound of protein after you start the re-feeding program again. Now they are fatter than when they started the diet in the first place and can't figure out what happened. What you are interested in is losing FAT, not weight!

This leads me to another question. Are you supposed to have FAT? Of course. You need fat for insulation, cushioning the body, femininity for women and reserve energy. Most exercise physiologists will agree that the acceptable level of body fat for a MALE is 15% or less and for WOMEN is 22% or less. <u>Unfortunately, the average MALE does not have 15%, he carries **26%** and the average FEMALE doesn't carry 22% she carries **31%**</u>.

The problem is that FAT hardly has a blood supply of its own, but your heart doesn't know it. Your heart pumps to mass. So, if you are carrying around an extra 10 pounds of FAT somewhere you don't want, your heart is trying to pump out blood, fuel and oxygen to feed it, and the capillary system may not go far enough or the blood vessels may not be elastic enough to handle the extra load put upon them. The result could be an explosion, away from the heart "Stroke", at the heart "Heart Attack".

Here is another important point: No matter what you are told, during the first 1-3 weeks of any diet 90 to 95% of the weight lost has nothing to do with fat. Your body is trying figure out what is going on and is holding onto the fat until it knows everything is okay; and that there will be enough energy coming in to sustain the bodily functions. Your body is losing only protein and water!

Remember you should be interested in losing FAT, not weight. Here is another interesting question to consider. Have you heard the word ANOREXIA? Why is it that I will measure an anorexic's body composition and find they are over-fat and yet literally starving to death? How can they be too fat under this circumstance?

Remember that every cell in your body is composed of some form of protein and regardless of what you are told, CARBOHYDRATES (fruits, vegetables, grains, beans, and legumes) are your primary source of energy. Fat is the highest potential source of energy, but unless trained to be used is the last one your body will utilize. Why? Because the anorexic is starving. The body thinks it is dying. Thus if any protein taken in it isn't used to build new cells; it is converted back to fat and stored for later. If carbohydrate is taken in, it isn't used to fuel the body; it is converted to Fat and stored for later. This Anorexic is over-fat and starving to death.

This brings me to another question. Why is it that WOMEN invariably outlive men? I have asked this question for years and never could get a good answer. Well I have it for you. It is because of the way we look. Let me tell any female reading this book what the "Ideal Man" is supposed to look like! The ideal man is supposed to have an 8-12 inch differential between his CHEST and his WAIST, in favor of his CHEST!

But for some reason, at about age 26 gravity starts to get the men and their CHESTS begin to move, downward and forward. Have you ever seen this? It is very serious. It is called "Furniture Disease". It is when a man's CHEST slides into his DRAWERS. It ends up in front of him and he can't stand up straight, so he tilts backwards. Then he coughs, sneezes, bends over to pick up a paper clip and herniates a disc in his back. He ends up with a $150,000 laminectomy (fusion of the lumber spine) and you ask him, "How did you hurt your back?" AND HE SAYS, "I SNEEZED!" IT HAPPENS EVERY DAY IN INDUSTRY.

But the question was, "Why is it that women outlive men?" A women's center of gravity is an inch and a quarter lower than a man's. So if her center of gravity falls, it tends to fall downward and backward. You get the dimpled effect often called "Cellulite". There really is no such thing. "Fat is fat", there is no cellular structure difference. Yet there are cellulite creams, salons, pills, wraps, rubs and centers dealing with something no one has in the first place. (See section: "The Cellulite Myth").

So there is your **Third Question**! Do you have something for Cellulite?

If they have something for it, get away from these people.

And the **Fourth Question** is: Where is the third-party, randomized, double-blind, crossover, peer-reviewed, published research to support the claims being made?

When you ask this question, you will eliminate 99% of everything on the market. Product manufacturers will say, "Clinical Studies say----". What clinical study? Where is it published? Where has it been presented? What doctor recommended this? Doctor of what? What are his or her credentials? Companies that advertise without this information are looking for people that are wearing a "Stupid Sign" across their chest.

What do the "research" terms mentioned above mean? Third-party means the research has not been done by the manufacturer of the product in question. Randomized means a computer decides which study group an individual is in, not the scientists conducting the study. Double-blind means neither the participants in the study nor the scientists conducting the study know who is taking the real thing and who is taking the placebo during the study. Crossover is actually a study within a study, as midway through the study the control and placebo groups are switched without participants' knowledge. Peer-reviewed indicates once the study is completed, a panel of experts review the results of the study for accuracy and will or will not recommend it for publication. Finally, published means the study will appear in a professional journal such as Medicine & Science in Sports & Exercise, The Journal of the American College of Cardiology, etc.

The Body Composition Ratio

The most important aspect of dieting in America, in my opinion, should be to alter the composition of your body, FAT vs. MUSCLE! This is measured as a percentage of your total body weight.

What is this percent of body fat? It is simply the amount of fat distributed inside your body and should be no more than 15-17% of your total weight for males and 22-24% for females. This is to reach the "Acceptable" category. To get into the "Athletic" category, males should be 11% or less and females 14% or less. It takes 3% to keep a male living and 7% to keep a female living.

Let me give you an example of what having a high percentage of body fat can mean to you. Have you ever run out of energy during the day? Particularly about 3 or 4 o'clock in the afternoon? You can hardly make it through the day. Then when you finally get home you are asleep by 6:30 p.m. or so in front of the television set.

What happened? Well, if you check this person's body fat you will most likely find it to be high. Fat absorbs the oxygen that they inhale and they run out of energy. This same person goes on a diet, loses weight, can't hold it and can't figure out why. Simple! They are losing things other than fat.

Checking body fat is a simple process. It can be done underwater in a "hydrostatic tank" or with "skinfold calipers". I do not make claims that fat loss is easy. In fact, there are countless millions of people all over the world that find it extremely difficult. For highly motivated individuals who take it upon themselves to lose fat weight, only about 20% will succeed. So you see, it isn't easy. It is one of the hardest things someone can do. However, your chances of succeeding are enhanced by the more information you have on how to lose fat weight safely and effectively.

When people begin approaching a diet they often think about their ultimate goal—"The Ideal Body Weight". But in reality there is no ideal body weight. Many people still go by actuarial tables published years ago by insurance companies, and this simply can't be done accurately. It makes more sense to talk about the composition of the body weight. What the scale tells you is how many pounds of weight you have gained or lost. It doesn't tell you what percentage of that weight loss, if any, was fat or what percent was other things.

What You Lose When You Diet

What other things do you think there might be? Some of the expendable components of the body are lost pretty readily when you go on a calorie-restricted diet. One of the easiest to lose is protein. Protein comes in many forms in the body, of which the largest is skeletal muscle. Protein is found in abundant quantities in muscle and is an expendable quantity; it is, in the economic exchange of energy in the body, one of three things to be consumed by the body.

One is FAT—the most desirable to lose. The second is protein and the third are a host of other things including vitamins, minerals and water. All of these can be expended and are in fact lost in proportion to one another in any kind of reducing plan, some more than others.

Losing weight, preferably fat weight, is actually easy to understand and complicated to put into practice. Simply, it means energy in vs. energy out. On one hand we have all the energy the body has available to it. This comes mostly in the form of food, but also energy reserve; stored energy that comes from various body components.

The most efficient form of stored energy in the body comes from fat. Fat is an unusual substance in that it doesn't do much. It sort of sits around and is not what is called "metabolically active". If you were to observe the day to day life of a fat cell you would find it very boring—it is simply an energy storage form. Under the microscope when you look at a fat cell, it just stares right back at you!

On the other hand, protein does a lot. Your muscles are the major energy expenders of the body. They are tremendously active, thus a tremendous user of energy. Under a microscope, when you look at a muscle cell, which contains a lot of protein, it looks like the 4th of July! At the same time, protein is a very poor storage form of energy. Fat then, is an excellent storage form but is difficult to liberate energy from because it is so inactive. You really have to stress the energy supply maximally to get fat to be used for energy purposes.

Another component that can be lost readily is water. Water, along with some of the more important vitamins and minerals in your body; particularly things like calcium, and other minerals found in unbelievably small quantities. These can be lost when the dieting regimen doesn't provide adequately in terms of these particular substances.

What happens when you diet to lose weight? First, all the energy that you take in has to be less than the body produces. SIMPLE! If the energy you are taking in is less than the body requires handling its basic workload, then it will need some sort of supplemental energy; the body absolutely requires it! So, what does your body do? It calls upon all of these expendable components and it doesn't do so in a very nice way.

For example, if fat is the best storage form of energy, you would think the body would use this source first when there is a caloric deficit; this is the basis of any diet. Regardless of what you hear, caloric deficit, that is, less calories taken in than you need is what is going to cause you to lose weight. There is no other way; it is a Law of Physics called thermodynamics. It is a big word that means that calories do count!

So, any diet to be effective has to be reduced in calories. When the body senses this caloric deficit, it will draw upon reserves. But it doesn't do it in an orderly and efficient way unless you maximize the chances for it to do so.

Starvation Diets—Don't Work!

So let's take a look at someone who decides to starve himself or herself, there is no energy coming in. Within 24 hours the body has used up all of its most efficient energy reserve. Energy reserve is basically carbohydrate. Carbohydrate is a sugar-like compound. Sucrose is a carbohydrate (table sugar). Ultimately carbohydrate comes down to one particular substance called glucose. Glucose is the immediate fuel reserve for the body to do its work. It is used constantly, especially by certain specialized parts of the body—one of which is the brain. The brain demands glucose. Glucose comes from dietary carbohydrate; what you eat (fruits, vegetables, grains, legumes, beans) or from artificial carbohydrate—other body components.

In reality, what dieting is all about is to cause the body to draw upon its resources to manufacture certain energy substances. The two energy sources that can be used are glucose (the carbohydrate) and another type of compound called a ketone. Ketones are provided by fat, they are the energy provided by fat.

The problem is that to make fat into a ketone is a big deal for the body chemically; it takes a long time. But during starvation all the reserve carbohydrate is gone after 24 hours. The body now makes decisions based upon absurd circumstances. It needs all this energy but isn't getting any, so it decides to divvy up whatever comes along according to certain priorities; and number one in priority in terms of energy utilization is Brain Cells.

Brain cells have an absolute requirement for carbohydrate (glucose). About 20% of the total population of brain cells cannot live without carbohydrate; they will not use anything else! So, fact number one is that your body is going to manufacture carbohydrate regardless. When it stops manufacturing it, guess what you are? DEAD—that's what!

How does your body make carbohydrate? Well, the body can make it in a number of ways. You can make it from fat, which would be ideal. You can make it from protein, and of these two choices, unfortunately the protein makes it more efficiently than fat does. So, given the correct set of circumstances the body will reject fat and say, "I'm going to use the PROTEIN since I can get the carbohydrate (glucose) much faster." And that's exactly what happens with starvation. You get losses almost immediately. Within 7 days up to 40% of any weight loss will be from protein.

Initially, if you looked at the first 7 days of someone that is totally starving, you would find the protein losses to be very great; the reason being that all of the brain cells want glucose. Finally, at the end of 7 days or so 80% of them have given up and say, "Okay, if you're going to be that way I'll use ketones." But that last 20% will not give up, they refuse. The body will continue to supply carbohydrate for the last 20% holdout. So that is what happens with starvation.

It also turns out that this is what happens when you are on a low calorie (less than 1000) type diet because it allows so few calories, which is basically the same as zero! I know it doesn't make much sense but it is true. In fact, you will lose equal amounts on a low calorie type of program, as you will by starving. After a very short period of time, the weight loss for someone who is on a total fast and someone on a very low calorie type program will be almost identical because the calories that are going in are immediately expended for the manufacture of whatever kinds of reserve protein the body can hold onto, which is basically nothing!

In fact, any low calorie diet that provides such a bare minimum of energy is basically a semi-starvation diet. For all intents and purposes the effect on your body is going to be the same; very dramatic losses of protein, some loss of fat—but the fat loss will be tremendously inefficient, and takes place very slowly.

It can actually be shown that you can put one group of people on a 1500-calorie per day diet, another on a 500-calorie per day diet, and if you compare the weight loss over the first 3 weeks, the diet group on the lower calories will lose more weight. Their scale will say they lost more weight. But if you look at their body composition, the group on the 1500-calorie per day diet has lost more fat.

And this is the KEY point. You don't want to lose skeletal muscle or smooth muscle; you don't want your liver, stomach or spleen to shrink in size, which they will do—very dramatically! You don't want your blood protein, which is responsible for immunity and blood coagulation to be dissipated because they are all expendable, they are protein! The body will chew them up just like it chews up other protein.

So the consequences of these dramatic, rapid weight loss programs that are tremendously restricted in calories are pretty impressive. Unfortunately, only a small percentage of it is actually coming from fat reserve. This is because you just can't push fat molecules too far. They will go just so far, so fast and that's it. This varies from person to person; each person is very specific as to the rate at which they are capable of dissolving or using body fat.

But for each individual there is an upper limit—they can't push themselves beyond this by any means. You can't take enzyme tablets that burn it up; you can't take little tablets that turn it into heat and don't store it as fat. You can't do anything like that. It is possible to lose about 3.3 pounds of actual fat in 7 days and that's it! So far medical technology and research have been unable to identify any way to speed up fat loss other than at the rate it wants to melt away by itself.

Any approach to weight loss must, therefore, be reasonable. It must be well balanced in terms of caloric intake. Figure out your minimum caloric intake needs by taking your best weight, the weight at which you feel most comfortable, and add a zero. This will give you a good estimate of your basal metabolic rate—your base caloric need.

A Balanced Program—That Works!

A perfectly balanced nutrition program meeting exact caloric requirements is recommended by most nutritionists. But why hasn't the 1500-calorie diet been successful if it is so conventional? Well, the problem is that it is very difficult to count calories that specifically. Have you ever tried to count calories? Is it easy? First, there is no uniformity on how things are prepared, so counting calories is ridiculous. To look up in a book and say "omelet" this many calories is ridiculous because it isn't true.

Traditionally, calorie counting, applying the principle of reduced calorie diets doesn't work. Second is the popular misconception provided by the traditionalist who says, "What is the energy cost of one pound of fat? What does it cost the body to buy one pound of fat?" Have you ever seen the number 3500 calories? One pound of fat = 3500 calories, so therefore if you take in 500 less calories per day times 7 days you get one pound of weight loss per week. Is this true? NO! Because if an individual stuck to that and reduced their caloric intake by 500 calories per day and they were very over-fat, they would lose more than one pound in a week, providing they are expending more than 500 calories in energy.

On the other hand, if someone only has to lose 1 pound or so, and they stuck to that program, they wouldn't lose a pound a week. Why? First of all, the energy cost of a pound of fat is different at the beginning of a diet than it is at the end—very different! This is because your body will automatically adjust that energy expenditure and will try to save your life. You see, when you start dieting, as I've said before, your body thinks you are trying to kill it! It thinks you are trying to commit suicide. And, it will make all kinds of adjustments—it will adjust energy expenditures up or down depending on what the circumstances are; it is a very, very fine tuned mechanism.

But realistically it is too simplistic to think that 3500 calories per pound is the ideal way to go. So what is the ideal diet? Well if there is no ideal weight is there such a thing as an ideal diet? Probably not for everyone, because if there were, the problem with over-fatness wouldn't be as great as it is!

But some general considerations do apply for any kind of approach to fat loss. One of the most important is that the diet should be nutritionally complete, because any diet that's not will be an inefficient diet. The body needs certain things in order to use chemical factories that are enzymes to get rid of fat. The body needs certain components of fuel to do that work, so if you are deficient in any of these you are not going to lose fat efficiently.

Secondly, it should be relatively easy for someone to implement, and that takes into account all kinds of considerations. How much is it going to cost me; am I going to some diet center and pay someone $400 per month and have them tell me not to eat 2 pounds of bacon with my eggs in the morning?—I can't do that! No one can do that! You can't put out that kind of money to have someone tell you you're too fat. People already know they are! These people give you a low calorie book and say "take this home—get this food and try to make some sense out of it".

So how much do you lose following this kind of program? You lose $400 dollars! How much fat do you lose? Who knows? Maybe none! Most people lose none on programs like this. So a good program has to be economical; it has to be convenient; it has to fit into some kind of lifestyle that you're used to, because if you disrupt your lifestyle what do you think your chances are that you're going to stick with it? Probably Zero!

One weight control program that I recommend that meets all of the requirements necessary for a medically and nutritionally sound program is the Juice Plus+® Program (outlined in Chapter Three). The advantages of the Juice Plus+® Program are that it fulfills all of these requirements: a) it is nutritionally complete, b) it is easy to implement into your lifestyle—it doesn't require that you do extraordinary things, c) it is inexpensive, and d) it is easy to mix up at home or take with you. I will describe this program more as we go along.

The third thing an "ideal diet" should have is opportunity. That opportunity should be used to re-educate yourself as to the kinds of things that led to your state of misfortune in the first place. And these considerations are an integral part of the Juice Plus+® Program because the program's philosophy of weight management is that you accomplish manipulating energy best in two ways: first, limiting the supply of energy through reasonable knowledge of what kinds of caloric considerations should be followed in your diet (The Nutripoints™ Program for Optimal Nutrition is recommended—again, more on this as we continue) and, number two, increasing the output side which is exercise.

"Hypokinetic Disease"

This brings me to another point. In the United States today the most common cause of over-fatness is not overeating. It is INACTIVITY! Sometimes called Hypokinetic Disease. In fact, if you look at groups of people in a systematic fashion you will constantly find that those who are over-fat, unless they suffer from some very rare medical condition (and don't get me wrong, there are people with genuine metabolic problems that cause them to be over-fat; but these are extremely rare), they simply don't expend enough energy. It has been looked at in all age groups from adolescence on up through old age, and the principal cause of over-fatness has been that energy expenditure is inadequate— INACTIVITY!

Increase Your Intensity!

On the other hand, some people are "moving" their body, but their "intensity" is not high enough to get the desired results.

Let me give you an example. After finishing a seminar one evening, a gentleman came up to see me; he was about 5' 8" inches tall and told me he weighed 350 pounds. He said he ate really good, which was pretty obvious, drank a lot of water, which is good, and walked 6 miles every day. I said, "If you do all these things how come you weight 350 pounds?" He said, "That's why I came up to see you—what's wrong with what I'm doing?"

I told him that his exercise *intensity* wasn't, in my opinion, high enough; I said, "Let me give you an example of how to raise your intensity. Take your sport coat off; when I say GO I want you to get to the other end of this room and back to me as fast as you can, without running—GO!"

When he got about half way to the other end of the room, you could actually hear him breathing hard. When he got back to me, he was gasping for breath. I said, "Don't stop, just slow down and continue walking around the room until you can breathe normally—I'll wait." It took him about 15 minutes to recover.

We repeated this task three times and each time it took him longer to recover. I told him, "You need to raise your exercise intensity! When you go for your next walk, instead of walking 6 miles, pick an object out in front of you, like a telephone pole, then see how fast you can get there (without running), slow down and keep walking until you recover, then repeat 5 or 6 times. You'll find amazing things will happen in a mile or less, instead of 6+ miles each day, simply because you have raised your intensity.

Give it a try, call me in 3 weeks and let me know what has happened; but I'll bet you'll probably be heavier in 3 weeks than you are now; but other good things will happen! Are you willing?" He said "I'll give it a try starting tomorrow!"

Three weeks later he called and said, "I'm 10 pounds heavier now than I was 3 weeks ago—what happened?" I said, "Before I tell you, what else has happened?" He answered saying, "I've lost significant inches off each thigh, my calves, waist and shoulder girth."

Why is this? Because muscle is heavier than fat, but takes up less space. For the first 3 weeks of this program, his body wasn't sure what was going on so his "body fat" stayed the same, actually waiting for him to quit, but his lean tissue increased. He actually got heavier and thinner at the same time. After 3 weeks his body said, "You're serious, I guess I don't need this extra fat; I'll let it go." I told him, "Keep using this program, at least on alternate days, for the next 6 weeks and see what happens."

He called after six more weeks saying he had lost 27 pounds (mostly fat) and was very excited about what was happening and what was going to continue happening. I congratulated him and said, "If you want continued positive success, you have to increase your *nutritional* intensity to match the increase in your *exercise* intensity." I suggested he use the Nutripoints™ program (see Nutrition section) to re-design his nutritional program and bridge the gap between his *current* nutrition level and *optimal* nutrition by adding Juice Plus+® to his program.

When you start any exercise program it is going to take somewhere between 3 and 12 weeks before you start seeing visible results. Positive things will be happening early in your training but many happen "inside out" before you notice them. Remember, there is no MAGIC pill. It's going to take hard work and patience—but I guarantee it will be worth it!

Timing of Meals—Key to Weight and Fat Loss

So what we would like to do in this program is engender some ideas that get people to realize that both sides of the equation do count. Energy intake is just as important as energy output and you really can't have one without the other. Because first of all, there are a number of people who are over-fat, not because they take in too many calories in a day, but because they take them in all at once. For example, the busy executive, someone who gets up in the morning and rushes out of the house to go to work, doesn't eat a thing all day long, comes back home and just piles 1600 calories (if he weighs 160 pounds) into one meal at dinner, then sits back, puts his feet up and relaxes. At this point the gastrointestinal tract is at its maximum point after a large meal (the feeling of complete lethargy!).

But this is the common problem that many people have. They don't actually overeat; if you look at their caloric intake it might be less than you and I, but they take it in all at one time. And what time of day do they take it in? At a time of day when they are least active; so their energy expenditure is totally out of proportion to their energy intake. And their metabolic system can sense this!

You can take someone who is eating 3000 calories per day and measure their basal expenditure of energy, and then start making them take all of them at night and you will find that within a very short period of time their body has sensed that its caloric intake is very different. So the body cuts back on its energy expenditure during the day because it knows that you are not going to take any food in. It literally senses that you are trying to do something bad to it, so it says, "Okay! You're not going to take any food in, fine; I'm going to lower the energy rate across the board so I don't need the food during the day."

Then, at night you get this tremendous wave of calories coming in when your basal metabolic rate is at its lowest rate. You have a double punch; first your body has sensed that your caloric input during the day is very low, so in an attempt to save you from certain suicide your body shuts its energy manufacturing centers down to an absolute low level.

So if you measure that person's energy output during the day you will find it will drop way off. Second, at night you dump in a whole bunch of calories and go right to bed where you don't expend any energy at all except what it takes to keep you alive. And this in itself will create a state of over-fatness.

So simple manipulation of your lifestyle if you have the opportunity to re-educate yourself about this can make a very big difference; and the addition of small increments of physical activity can have astronomical effects on the rate at which your body uses energy, even at rest.

Let's use an example here: There are two people, both weighing

160 pounds; one is 12% body fat, the other is 20% body fat. If you look at the energy expenditure of both these people at rest (totally asleep), the one with 12% body fat will be burning up far more calories per hour than the one with 20% body fat.

Because, remember, the more fat you have, the less metabolic activity is going on. Fat doesn't do anything; it just sits there. Basically it has no blood supply. It doesn't require any exchange of chemicals to do its job of sitting around. So, if your body weight is distributed in a large percentage of fat, your metabolic activity will be very low. In choosing a diet or an approach to weight loss, you want to be selective. You want to attack FAT—not just weight! Why then do we feel that the Juice Plus+® Program is so good?

The Importance of Protein

First of all, the PROTEIN! Protein is a very efficient user of energy. In fact, one measure of the efficiency of a compound in terms of promoting caloric expenditure is to see how much work the body has to do just to get it inside, because this requires energy too. When you eat something, especially protein, energy systems are activated from your intestinal tract in the blood stream. Juice Plus+ Complete®, a highly nutritious meal replacement drink which is part of the Juice Plus+® Program, uses up a significant number of calories just getting into your system—that's pretty good! What it means is that this protein is used very effectively for metabolism.

The other thing is that it promotes the replenishment of those protein stores that are being attacked by the body's constant need for carbohydrate production. Remember, if you are losing weight your body has this irreducible requirement for this carbohydrate. It is going to use some protein and some fat at different rates. It uses protein more effectively than fat and so you have to do something to get back the protein the body is going to expend. If you don't, a lot of the weight loss is going to be in protein.

The key point here is that once you start the re-feeding period (going off your diet) your body will immediately regain the lost protein. You can easily understand then why someone who is on a very low calorie type diet for a long period of time says the very week they went back on their regular diet, they gained 15 pounds back. And this is a conservative estimate. Some people gain back 20 pounds in one week because they gain back 5 pounds of protein and 15 pounds of water with it. The water comes back by hook or crook; it has to, it's a chemical law.

Measuring Protein Quality

The "quality" of the protein is also important. How do we measure it? Protein Efficiency Ratio (PER) was for many years the standard for evaluating protein ingredients. This procedure has been replaced by the Protein Digestibility Corrected Amino Acid Score (PDCAAS). This score (or value) is determined by taking into account how digestible a protein is, in addition to comparing its essential amino acid profile to the essential amino acid profile needed for growth by a young child age 2-5 years. This value is never greater than 1.0 but it can be less than one.

For a beverage, the FDA (Food and Drug Administration) considers a product to be an "excellent" source of protein if it contains more than 20% DV (Daily Value) per cup and is considered a "good" source of protein if it contains between 10-19 DV per cup; based upon a 2000 calorie per day diet.

What does this mean in reference to Juice Plus+ Complete® mentioned earlier? It means the rating for Juice Plus+ Complete® is better than good, it is <u>excellent</u>! One serving equals one cup and Juice Plus+ Complete® has a 25% DV (Daily Value) per serving; excellent by anyone's standards. It contains a vegetable protein blend including soy protein, tofu powder, and chickpea powder. The advantages of the soy protein used in Juice Plus+ Complete® over other proteins are the isoflavone and phyto-estrogen benefits. These phytonutrients (plant-based nutrients) provide cardiovascular disease benefits according to the FDA. Also, soy contains no lactose and is a vegetable protein, which provides many health benefits over animal or milk-based proteins.

There is also Lactobacillus acidophilus in Juice Plus+ Complete® which is a very beneficial probiotic, generally referred to as a "gut friendly bacteria" (there are no negatives with these bacteria). It contains a blend of fibers including oat fiber, rice bran, citrus pectin, apple fiber and other dietary fibers. It has a blend of both simple (such as fructose) and complex (such as fructooligosaccharides) carbohydrates for a smooth rise in, and maintenance of blood glucose levels. And, there are no ingredients in Juice Plus+® Complete (or Juice Plus+® Capsules, another part of the program which is a whole food-based concentrate of fruits and vegetables) that would cause an Olympic athlete or any other athlete to fail a drug test!

This, in my opinion, is why it is called Juice Plus+ Complete®. It is a perfectly balanced meal-replacement that is rated at the top of the list, compared to others (see p. 233, 247), by Dr. Roy Vartabedian, author of **Nutripoints,** and co-author of this book.

What About Fat?

Here is another point. It just so happens that ridding yourself of all fat in your diet is a bad thing to do, because like many other nutrients, certain fats are absolutely required by the body. Fat, although the storage form does nothing, in the non-storage form it does a lot chemically, especially in the absorption of vitamins. Many vitamins can only be absorbed in the presence of certain fats; if you don't have the fat in your diet, you don't get the vitamins—they are not absorbed. The intestines will wash them out—they won't be picked up by the bloodstream at all.

Did you know that unsaturated fatty acids also have a little enzyme system in them that helps break down storage fat? In the actual conversion of storage fat to energy the body will use active unsaturated fatty acids to help break it down.

The stomach gets rid of fat very slowly. This is what keeps you full and satisfied after a high-fat meal. It takes 3 1/2 to 4 hours for the stomach to empty a high fat meal (10 grams per hour). This means that for 3 1/2 to 4 hours various small quantities of fat are being released into the small intestine; getting into the bloodstream where they elevate your blood sugar. One feature of a good fat loss program would be to contain foods high in fiber which slow down the release of glucose in the blood stream simulating this effect of fat.

One part of the Juice Plus+® Program I like in relation to this point are "Juice Plus+ Thins®", which are flavorful, chewable bite-sized wafers containing various high-quality fibers and slow-release sweeteners. These give you the practical advantage of acting as a hunger suppressant, because they help sustain blood sugar levels over a period of time. They can be eaten 15-20 minutes before a meal or in-between meals. So after you take the Juice Plus+ Thins®, your blood sugar level will be relatively constant and you are less likely to be hungry.

Multiple vitamins and minerals are also very important in a fat loss program, since you will be restricting calories; but the problem with taking a separate vitamin/mineral supplement is that current research says they work much better when they are in their natural state (in food) rather than being fragmented. With the Juice Plus+® Program you have the highest Nutripoint-rated type of concentrate available. Juice Plus+® Capsules, a key part of the program, contain whole food-based concentrates, taken from 15 different high quality fruit and vegetable juice and pulp powders and the bran from two grains (see Dr. Vartabedian's ratings on p. 244, 246). The Juice Plus+ Complete® drink also contains some of the powders contained in the capsules.

Supervised Medical Programs

"Medically Supervised Dramatic Weight Loss" is a semi-starvation diet using three meal-replacement formula servings per day called "Protein-Modified Fasting". Have you ever heard of this? It is very complicated and we won't go into detail; but one former example of this type of diet was the "Alpha II Ultra Diet". It said right on the label "This is a Protein-Sparing Modified Fast". All we really want to tell you about this type of program is that they are effective for people who are what is called "morbidly obese". That is, people who are so overweight that they stand a very good chance of having a horrendous medical problem develop directly from their state of over-fatness. Many of these people, because of their extreme obesity, are at risk for their very lives. So in some circumstances it is justifiable to have these people lose tremendous amounts of weight very quickly.

For example, if you wanted to prepare someone for an urgent operation, a Protein-Sparing Modified Fast is appropriate. They are appropriate ONLY, and we emphasize ONLY (because certain commercial products will tell you otherwise) when followed by someone who is an expert in this type of metabolic manipulation; and this excludes almost all General Practitioners instantly. This is a very technical, highly complicated process that requires absolute day to day follow-up by a very experienced physician. You cannot read on a label how much of this or that to take and expect to be safe on this type of program. Most people who need to lose body fat do not need a Protein Sparing Modified Fast. In addition, it is very expensive because you can't do it on your own.

So, the answer is a more conventional approach with a modest reduction in calories such as in the Juice Plus+® Program. The Juice Plus+® Program is basically a conventional low-fat, low-calorie diet disguised as a formula weight-management program; except only one of the three meals replaced by a formula (always check with your doctor before beginning any weight-loss program). It uses low-calorie Juice Plus+ Complete® in place of a meal or as a between-meal snack, once or twice a day. It happens to work as an excellent fat loss program. It is the type of program you can easily incorporate into your eating habits; it is a means by which you can regulate body composition fairly directly and easily without worry that you are going to engender all kinds of health problems. It serves as a very simple, useful way to intake a specific number of wholesome calories each day and modify your body fat. It is also a program that people, once they achieve the kind of fat loss they want, can use as a regular dietary addition.

How Low Is Too Low-Calorie

What is a low calorie diet? Probably less than 800-1000 for even the most sedentary people. So any diet of calories less than this will be a Ketosis-producing diet. You will have a lot of these ketones floating around because the energy deficit is so great that you are losing large amounts of weight very rapidly.

What happens to the ketones in the blood? Well, ketones are acids, so if too many of them buildup in the bloodstream you can suffer a very severe metabolic problem called ACIDOSIS! Too much acid in the bloodstream! Some of the ketones are used as primary fuel; for example, exercising muscle can use ketones for energy. Those that are used for energy end up as alcohol in the blood and are disposed of by various means. The ketones remaining are flushed through the kidneys at a very high rate, which is the reason that any ketosis producing diet is extremely dehydrating. This is because when these ketones get flushed out of the kidney they drag large amounts of water with them.

So, on a balanced program, like the Juice Plus+® Program, how do you get rid of the fat? In this plan adequate carbohydrate is provided to fuel the body's brain cells so there is always enough glucose around. Because of this, the fat can be metabolized at a slower rate and the ketones will then provide the fuel for muscle. And this is why it is advantageous to provide an exercise program along with your nutrition program; because the more your muscles exercise the more efficient they are at using fat for energy. They can literally tune themselves up.

For example, you are starting a vigorous exercise program; let's say riding a bike at 15 mph constantly for one hour. If you are not a trained athlete you will find that virtually the entire energy supply will come from carbohydrate. If you are a trained athlete, the first 15 minutes of energy will come from carbohydrate, but the last 45 minutes will come from fatty acid (triglyceride or ketones), and this is a tune-up job. It's one of those automatic things that your body's metabolism can do to help regulate energy balance.

This is the reason that tuned up musculature is a much better machine than flabby or un-toned muscle. But, fat loss will reach a maximum in most people of 2-3 pounds per week. That's about the fastest at which it can be broken down and pumped into the system for use; you really can't exceed that. So if you are achieving fat loss of 3 pounds per week you are really doing a good job.

Most people don't do that. In fact, any diet when first started will initiate weight loss through loss of water. The more fat you have to lose, and the heavier you are, in the first 1-2 weeks of your program the weight loss will be artificial; it will come from large amounts of water loss. But you want to avoid, in addition to the water loss (which comes invariably), the loss of protein with it; because if you are losing predominantly protein you aren't doing yourself any good. When you lose protein you are losing the tissue that is metabolically active; you are losing the material that provides energy expenditure.

So the weaker you get, the less caloric expenditure there will be per day and, the less efficient your weight loss will be. Everyone who has studied this has shown that weight loss becomes less efficient with progress through a low calorie diet. Your body will automatically adjust so that your actual fat utilization will slow down markedly. This is why many people who lose tremendous amounts of weight initially will reach a plateau, and they virtually eat nothing and lose nothing. The body has adjusted and now instead of losing water it is conserving it.

Most people can't put up with this kind of program because they are so unpalatable and ridiculously rigid. Less than 800 calories is a ketosis producing diet. It will produce a state of ketosis fairly rapidly and problems ensue: dehydration which can lead to very severe drops in blood pressure, especially when you change posture (laying down to standing up), extreme protein loss which is replenished very rapidly when you start eating normally again; a form of arthritis called "GOUT" –the most excruciating, acute arthritis there is, and severe vitamin-mineral deficiency.

All of these things are common in extreme low calorie programs. They are much less efficient than the moderate and balanced programs like Juice Plus+® Program described. People on extreme low calorie diets lose more weight, but they don't lose more fat—they lose less fat! So let me reiterate a few points as we finish this section:

1. I recommend that you stay away from low-calorie diets, and "quick fixes" that are advertised with no substantial, published research to support their claims.

2. Body fat is more important than body weight. The acceptable level for males is 15% or less and for females 22% or less. It takes 3% body fat to keep a male living and 7% for a female. Eleven percent or less is the Athletic category for a male and 14% or less for a female. Remember that muscle is heavier than fat but takes up less space. So you can actually get on the correct type of exercise program and gain muscle weight while at the same time losing inches.

3. A sound "fat" loss program should include exercise as an important element (See Chapter Two). Exercise burns up calories, but in addition one of the biggest benefits is maintenance or improvement of lean body mass.

4. If you cut your caloric intake down without a corresponding

increase in energy expenditure your metabolism slows down to compensate. The result—unsuccessful fat loss.

5. There are seven groups of nutrients: protein, carbohydrate, fat, minerals, vitamins, fiber, and water. In addition, there are essential enzymes, and thousands of plant nutrients which are virtually undiscovered but have positive effects known as phytochemicals or phytonutrients. These are found primarily in whole, unprocessed foods and whole food concentrates.

6. Water is the most essential of all nutrients. We can live only 4 days without water. We should drink 2-3 glasses of water over and above the amount suggested by thirst alone. To test your proper level of water intake check the color of your urine from day to day. A urine color darker than a light straw color would suggest the need for greater fluid intake. Clinical studies have shown that water supplementation, 2-3 large glasses with each meal, can result in a one pound per week weight loss without any diet, exercise or pills. (See "Maintaining the Right Fluid Balance" in section following.)

7. The human body may obtain energy from 4 sources: carbohydrate, fat, protein and alcohol. Carbohydrates are by far the best; next is protein if it can be efficiently converted to a carbohydrate by the toned body. Alcohol is an especially poor source since it cannot even supply energy to muscles; fat is difficult to get moving and research has clearly linked excess fat consumption to a number of serious diseases including heart disease and cancer. Thus, carbohydrates and protein are the two cornerstones of a successful program. We have a minimum requirement of 23 grams of protein each day, providing that the protein has a high biological value

with the proper balance of amino acids. In actual practice it is recommended that we consume about 50 grams of protein every day.

8. Modern living gets in the way of eating wisely. The U.S. Department of Agriculture has reported that one of every two Americans is nutritionally deficient. This means that at least 50% of our population is malnourished; and the numbers continue to grow. Not because of poverty but because of poor food choices and consuming foods of poor nutritional quality. Due to chemical fertilizing, food processing, prolonged shelf life, and the fact that people eat imitation fast foods and fast food snacks drink, alcohol, coffee, soft drinks, etc., our nutritional status is further degraded.

9. If you ate a fully nutritious diet and your body was able to assimilate all the essential vitamins, minerals and enzymes it needed and, you could take in the recommended 9-13 servings of fresh raw fruits and vegetables each day you probably would not need to consider taking a food supplement to make up the difference. Since nobody is perfect and most of us don't even come close, we should all consider taking some type of supplementation; especially during a low-calorie regime (see Chapter Four for recommendations).

10. A good diet includes all of the necessary vitamins/minerals, amino acids, carbohydrate, protein and fatty acids that the body needs. A great recommendation for a balanced diet would be the "Nutripoints™ Program for Optimal Nutrition" by Dr. Roy Vartabedian, Dr.P.H. This program (which teaches you which are the most nutrient dense foods—see

www.Nutripoints.com for more information), combined with the benefits of Juice Plus+® can lead to Ultimate Nutrition for you and your family.

11. The Juice Plus+® Program and the Nutripoints™ Program described in this book are supported by Designs for Fitness because they are nutritionally, biologically and medically sound, and are supported by peer-reviewed, published research that cannot be denied. They are safe and sensible ways to change your body inside out, and produce lasting fat loss. So there you are—you have the facts! What then is the next step? If you are serious about improving your health and increasing your nutritional intensity, start now and keep reading!

MAINTAINING THE RIGHT FLUID BALANCE

Water and the Body

Water makes up an average of 70% of total body mass. Muscle contains 72-78% water, whereas only 50% of the body fat (adipose tissue) is water.

About 62% of total body water is intracellular (inside cells) and 38% occurs extracellularly (outside cells) in plasma, lymph, and other fluids outside the cell. Water provides structure and form to the body and plays a crucial role in temperature regulation. Exercise in hot weather greatly increases the body's water requirement, and in extreme conditions, fluid needs increase 5 or 6 times above normal.

There is some body water loss every day, and after only a few days of severe dehydration can result in death.

Water and Weight Control

If you don't take in an adequate amount of water, you will likely find it impossible to achieve control over your weight. What this means is 10-12 eight ounce glasses of WATER per day, plus eight more ounces for every 25 pounds you are overweight. This is the basic requirement for healthy living. Unfortunately, not many people drink as much water as they need.

Increasing your water intake can cure many problems of weight control. Constipation, nausea, and headaches can all be helped with this, the greatest nutritional supplement in the world. WATER!

First, by not drinking enough water, you can actually cause your body to retain fluid. Four or five cups of coffee in the morning, a glass of wine at lunch, another cup of coffee or a soft drink in the afternoon, a cocktail before dinner and a couple of cups of coffee after dinner isn't what I'm talking about.

People who drink like this say they are always thirsty. Their body is being deprived of the water needed to keep itself healthy and it reacts by retaining almost every drop of the tiny bit it is allowed by your stopping at the water cooler once or twice each day. The body often gets puffy and swollen as a result. The extra weight you think of as fat may not be fat at all.

Other Fluids Count...Don't They?

Wine, gin, coffee, tea, fruit juices, and soft drinks are all fluids, but they don't have the same chemical properties as ordinary water. Alcohol and soda pop contain too much sugar, so to a lesser extent do fruit juices. The caffeine in coffee and tea is bad for your heart and blood pressure. Even diet soda contains sodium, which contributes to water retention. Cut down on coffee, drink sugarless drinks if you like them, but most importantly, drink 10-12 eight ounce glasses of water daily.

Side Effects of Low Water Intake

Restricting your water can promote fat deposits. Your body uses water as the major component of blood to transport nutrients and wastes. A lack of water in the system can cause fats and other toxins that are normally disposed of, to remain in your body—including that dimpled fat commonly referred to as "cellulite".

Your kidneys have a difficult time processing contaminated water, so your liver has to detoxify it. This means your liver can't do its main task, which is to process your blood and help break down fat. Thus, as you store water, the fat you eat can be stored in fat cells instead of being broken down in the liver. You become bloated, waterlogged, and obese.

Finding the Right Fluid Balance

The good news is that it is easy to solve this problem. An 8 oz. glass of water isn't very large. Keep it on your desk and keep refilling it. Don't go by the water cooler without taking a sip, thirsty or not. Keep a glass on your night stand and drink when you first get up.

Dieters and non-dieters alike must establish a "fluid balance" where water going into the body approximately equals the amount being excreted. When you reach this balance point, you will see the incredible difference water can make in your weight control program. Pounds and inches begin to disappear.

Trying to solve the problem of fluid retention by drinking less water only aggravates matters, because it (retention) occurs even when you drink no water. If you don't drink more water after salty food, your body pulls water from your intestines and bowel to dilute the extra sodium. If you drink more water, you force stored water out of your body through the kidneys.

How Much is Too Much?

You don't have to worry about drinking too much water—it is virtually impossible! Any excess will be urinated and/or sweated out.

Diuretics for Weight Loss?

What about diuretics? Diuretics force stored water out of your body. The problem is that your body perceives this as a lack of necessary water and stores whatever is available. So unless you are drinking enough water, diuretics won't usually solve the problem of retention. Diuretics can also cause constipation by draining water from the colon in order to distribute it around your body, because not enough water is available. Thus, without enough water in the colon, your stools can become dry and hard.

Start Now—Increase Gradually

I suggest you give water a chance. Only with an adequate supply of clean, fresh, life-giving water (nowadays purified or filtered is best), can your body's systems function in a way that keeps you healthy.

If you are unaccustomed to drinking water, this chart will help you comfortably increase your water consumption.

DAY	WATER	DAY	WATER
1	4-8oz. glasses	8	8-8oz. glasses
2	5-8oz. glasses	9	8-8oz. glasses
3	5-8oz. glasses	10	9-8oz. glasses
4	6-8oz. glasses	11	9-8oz. glasses
5	6-8oz. glasses	12	10-8oz. glasses
6	7-8oz. glasses	13	11-8oz. glasses
7	7-8oz. glasses	14	12-8oz. glasses

ARE YOU READY TO GET STARTED?

Whether you realize it or not, fitness and happiness have a lot in common. For instance, if you feel good, if you have a good self-image, it's easier to get up in the morning, you become more productive and everything tends to go better for you.

In reality your body needs three things:

1. It needs **rest** - and we usually get plenty.
2. It needs **fuel** - and we tend to over-fuel
3. It needs **exercise** - and we tend to under-exercise.

There are five reasons why people don't exercise. I think the number one problem is that the average person says, "I don't have time!" They will simply not spend 45 minutes to 1 1/2 hours per day exercising. The answer to this problem is: what will they do, at least 3 days per week, for the rest of their lives? We are talking about habit! You can't store fitness.

The second excuse is convenience. Exercise has to be convenient.

The third excuse, "I get bored doing the same thing over and over. As an example, if you start jogging 1 mile today, a year from now you might have to jog 6 miles to get the same result.

The fourth excuse is, "I get sore." The older you get, the sooner you get sore, the longer it lasts, and the more miserable you are. Incidentally, the biggest three days in the history of exercise are January 2nd, 3rd and 4th. This is the New Year resolution!

But the "key" excuse is, "I'm not motivated!" It's interesting to note that 80% of people you know don't care about your fitness problems and your lack of motivation; the other 20% are glad you are in worse shape than they are!

What does it take to have a successful fitness program?

First, you must educate yourself about what fitness is, and know your personal needs. Next, you must care about the way you look and feel—this is your motivation! Next, you have to "activate"—find a program that eliminates your excuses for not exercising and gives maximum results in the shortest amount of time. Finally, you evaluate your progress, which leads to continued motivation.

What is the average man interested in relative to fitness?

1. Living longer
2. His bad back—more than 84% of all Americans have back problems.
3. Arm strength
4. Waistline
5. Flexibility

What is the average woman interested in?

1. Back of the arms sagging—first sign of aging!
2. Bust line control and firmness.
3. Waistline
4. Hips and thighs
5. Inner and back part of the legs.

How can I motivate myself to get started?

Go into your bedroom, shut and lock the door behind you, turn on all the lights, take off all your clothes, stand in front of a full length mirror and see if you like what you see. Then allow 15 minutes for trauma to set in and now you're ready to go to work! You see, it doesn't matter what I want you to do, it only matters what you want to do.

Some simple tests for motivation:

Know something about your heart: how many times does it beat per minute? To find out, locate your pulse, using two fingers, either on the carotid artery on your neck or on the thumb side of your wrist. Count the number of heartbeats you feel for 6 seconds and add a zero. This represents your resting heartbeat at this moment. If you could drop this number by 10 beats per minute you save 14,000 heartbeats per day. This one factor could significantly extend your life expectancy.

Testing for strength! (Make sure you check with your physician before doing any of these tests). Can you do 10 push-ups in 10 seconds? If not, you don't have enough strength (in my opinion) in your upper body. How about abdominal crunches? Can you do 10 in 10 seconds? If you can't, your abdominal muscles are too weak.

Testing for flexibility. Don't try to compare your flexibility to that of anyone else. The important thing is where are you now and where do you finish. Check your low back, hip, hamstring, calf flexibility by sitting on the floor, legs straight out in front of you, toes up. Place one hand on top of the other and see if you can outreach your toes without discomfort; do not try to over-reach or bounce. If you can't at least reach your toes, you don't have enough lower body flexibility. By improving this factor you reduce the risk of lower back injury and hamstring pulls.

Upper body flexibility test. Place your hands on your hips with your index fingers on the hip bones. Squeeze your elbows together behind you and have someone measure the distance between them (inside to inside). The closer they go together (10" or less is very good) the more flexibility you have in the shoulder girdle. This helps reduce problems of stress headaches, pinched nerves and other problems.

Do you know someone who begins to run out of energy about 3:00 p.m. in the afternoon? They can barely get through the day and by 6:00 or 7:00 p.m. are asleep in front of the TV set. Two things have happened. Number one, they aren't strong enough to get through the day, and number two, their percentage of body fat is too high. As a result, the oxygen normally used by the body for energy gets absorbed by the fat in their body and they run out of energy. The only way to drop this % body fat is through exercise.

People often get involved in some kind of quick-fix diet and lose a lot of weight over a short period of time; but they can't maintain this new weight because, although their weight is less, their % body fat (relationship of fat to muscle) is the same. A good nutritional program is almost worthless without a good exercise program. You can have a body fat test done at your local health club, YMCA or university (exercise physiology department).

MOTIVATION FOR ULTIMATE SUCCESS

I want to try to do one of the most difficult things there is in life. I want to MOTIVATE you! If any of you know anything about motivation you know it is probably the hardest thing to do with a human being. How does a parent, for example, motivate his or her child? How does a coach motivate his or her team? How does a businessperson motivate his or her employees to do the things they ought to do? How does a preacher motivate a congregation?

When you begin to think about it, you realize that this is one of the hardest things that there is in life—to motivate somebody! And yet you and I both know it's the difference. For every one Olympic Champion there are 100,000 boys or girls who could be Olympic Champions. For every great salesperson; for every artist or painter or great professional leader in any capacity there are 100,000 people who could have been great, the difference is motivation. I can't even tell you what motivation is because it is difficult to define. It's something that just happens to a person—and they begin to act!

Like the track coach who had four boys on his relay team and they weren't putting out the way he thought they should. So he substituted, for the baton, a loaded stick of dynamite; and as the third boy handed this loaded stick of dynamite to the fourth boy who, running like mad, blazed down the straightaway into the tape. The coach was there with his stopwatch and nudged his assistant coach and said, "I told you those guys could run that in under 3 minutes!" Well that's motivation!

That's what I would like to do for you. I want to motivate you. I want to get you to act. I want to get you to use your abilities. I'm confident there is someone reading this right now that is capable of great things in life, and if I can just motivate you, I'm sure you can do what you ought to do.

So I'm going to speak out of the world I know the best, the world of athletic competition, borrowing from the sports world some wonderful stories, believing that out of these experiences you can see the crisis in your own life. You can see a simple answer to your own life; you can see the kind of emotion and drive that you need motivate yourself. And the first thing I want to say is this: **there comes a time in the sports world and in life when you've got to take a chance**. When you've got to put your neck out so to speak on the block. When you have to take a tremendous chance, you don't know all the answers but you give yourself to something, believing you can pull it off.

Now I'm not talking about a wild gamble like people sitting in casinos at slot machines or buying a lottery ticket waiting for some lucky break to change their life. I don't mean that kind of gamble. I mean where you put yourself into it, when you do something about it. An intelligent risk where you use your mind and give your life to something! Well the sports world rings with this kind of phenomenon.

Take professional football players, these guys, the seconds ticking away and they're behind in a ball game. A quarterback will go back and hit a receiver with a 50 or 60 yard pass in the end zone in the last remaining seconds to win the game. These players make the game so exciting because they are used to risk. They take the chance!

I think of the great golfer Arnold Palmer. A young reporter asked him once why he took a 10 on a hole in the Los Angeles Open and lost the championship. He asked Palmer, "Why didn't you play it safe?" Arnold Palmer replied, "Let me tell you something, son, you don't win big championships by playing it safe!" He said, "If I'm behind a tree I go through the tree. I found out there is a 50/50 chance you can go through that tree. When I go up to the ball I can't think to myself I've got to play it safe; that I might hook it or slice it. I've got to hit that shot precisely where I want it to go. You can't win big championships, son, by taking it easy; you've got to go for it!"

This is why this guy could put 4 or 5 birdies together under pressure in the last few holes to win a tremendous tournament. It is also why Arnold Palmer is considered to be one of the greatest golfers of all time. Why? Because he took the chance!

I submit to you that this is a reality we are going to have to live with in America. We live in an age of risk. It isn't easy. You can't play it safe; you can't just fall on the ball. We've got to use our imagination; we've got to reach out! I think of the famous Astronaut John Glenn. Just before he went up into outer space the first time a reporter asked him, "John, what are you going to do if your retro-rockets don't go off?" John Glenn looked at this guy, smiled and said, "You know, it's going to spoil my whole day." Of course the retro-rockets might not go off, but that's why men and women do great things—they take the chance!

America was built on this kind of psychology; people who left the security of the old shores and came to America because they took a chance on liberty. They died before they were 30, they fought for their lives, they half starved to death, but these men and women were willing to take the chance, the supreme chance of life itself—for <u>liberty</u>! Our country, our economics were built on this kind of philosophy, where men would lose everything and begin again. They would build a great industry; they'd lose it and build another one. That's why we have the greatest economy in the world!

We are bartering this away in this myopic socialism which says, "Don't take a chance; we'll take care of you. Let us plan your life from birth to the grave. You don't have to take any risks, the State is the answer to all your problems; the State will take care of you." We're bartering away the most precious thing we have in America today— OUR FREEDOM! Well, you can't have freedom without risk; you can't have progress without risk, you've got to be willing to take a chance.

But before you think I'm just talking politics, can I tell you the greatest risk ever taken in the history of the universe is when GOD made a man, put him on the earth, gave him a mind and a will and said, "Now live your own life, think your own thoughts". When GOD did that he took the supreme chance on human beings. I don't know about you but I'm here today because my parents, Ellsworth and Anna May Medina, believed in me when not many other people did.

I submit to you that there isn't a person of greatness but for what someone has taken a chance on his or her life. You can't escape risk in life. Marriage is a risk, the vocation you select is a risk, and in the international situation in which we find ourselves today we are going to have to live with risk. You can't beat those who are trying to destroy us by playing it safe, by a policy of containment; you've got to take chances!

Number two - **you must expect to fail**. I know this is a hard one to say to anyone, "You've got to fail, it's impossible to live without failing." Of course we like the opposite; we like to pick up a book on "How to be a Success."

Everyone wants to succeed. But what most books forget is the hard reality that in order to succeed you've got to fail. Failure is the road to success! I think it is probably 75% failure for every 25% success. Professional baseball players that step into the batter's box—don't they make outs 3 out of 4 times? They only hit safely about one out of every four times. It is the superlative player who goes much beyond that. We like to talk about the guy that hits home runs, but you know they strike out about 3 times for every one home run they hit. You look at the lives of these great athletes in sport and you realize they wallow through failure in order to get the dramatic moment.

About 25% of the people take responsibility regarding life; 75% will just drift along in mediocrity, they won't seize their opportunities, they won't do what they have to do. You've got to expect failure!

Many years ago I had the opportunity to watch one of the world's greatest sprinters, Frank Budd, blaze into the tape in 9.2 seconds, the 100-yard dash during the National Track & Field Championships in New York. The crowd was roaring its approval and Frank Budd was so happy. He was being interviewed by Bob Richards who asked, "It's a little bit different than Rome, isn't it?"

Very few people knew what he was talking about when he asked that question. In Rome the year before at the Olympic Games, Frank Budd had failed to get the baton to Ray Norton (my former teammate on the San Jose State College football team), his teammate in the relay.

He had wavered for a split second and during the waver Ray Norton went out of the exchange area. As a result the Americans lost four Gold Medals and a World Record.

In the roar of the crowd Frank Budd said this: "Bob, you have to go through Rome to appreciate a moment like this." A rather profound statement for a young man 20 years old. But do you see what he is driving at? You have to go through failure before you can even appreciate success. The people who want success after success after success, what they fail to realize is that they wouldn't appreciate it if they had it.

You have to experience failure before success has meaning. It was once put beautifully when someone said "Failure is GOD'S shock treatment, designed to bring a man or woman to a new realization of themselves!" Don't be afraid of failure. It's the process by which you get to the goal of victory and success.

Thirdly, and this one fits in with the other aspects of motivation, **you will be as big as you think you can be**. I know this sounds like a sweeping generalization. You say to me, "You mean I can be anything I want to be?" I say to you, you can! Before you deny me, let me tell you a few sports stories of what kids have done that seemed impossible.

Bob Richards, former Olympic Track and Field Champion, tells of the time he was in Champaign, Illinois giving a speech about the Olympic Games and said, "Who knows but what there is an Olympic Champion right here in the auditorium." He didn't really think much about it, signed a few autographs and left after the speech.

Two years later he went to Rome, Italy for the Olympic Games and watched kids battling for Gold Medals. He watched this kid from America named Mulligan. He didn't know what town in America Mulligan was from, but Mulligan was battling this swimmer from Australia. There was hardly a molecule of water between them, the roar of the crowd, lactic acid in their muscles, these guys tired—worn out; six yards to go—then four. In the last yard Mulligan reached out to barely beat this kid from Australia. Bob Richards, who was doing the commentary on this race, was so excited he ran down, threw his arm around Mulligan's shoulder and said, "That was tremendous!" This big old kid looked up at Bob and said, "Did you know that I was from Champaign, Illinois?"

Bob said he almost fell in the pool. That boy, what Bob Richards had said superficially—BELIEVED! Two years later he was the Olympic Champion. Do you see what I mean? You can be as big as you think you can be. He thought of himself as an Olympic Champion, two years later he was an Olympic Champion.

Let me tell you another one: Bob Richards was in Long Beach, California and as a minister had a church down there. He would go around to Sunday school classes talking about the great champions he once knew. Well, in a little class of girls 9-10 years of age, he was talking about some great tennis champions and a little 10-year-old girl jumped up in front of him and said, "Bob, I want to be a great tennis champion!"

Bob was actually embarrassed for this little girl and put his hand on her head and said, "Billie, I sure hope you can be a champion," and eased the way for her to sit down, thinking it was just an impulsive moment. Imagine his surprise when he picked up a newspaper and read that Billie Jean Moffett of Long Beach, California was the fourth ranking amateur tennis player in the World! Imagine his surprise when she scored one of the biggest upsets in Wimbledon Tennis History when along with her Doubles partner she won the Doubles Championship of the World. You see, she was as big as her challenge. This little curly haired girl got a dream and she began to reach out for it.

People are as big as they think they can be. Bob Richards made this personal reference when he said, "In Oslo, Norway I went over the crossbar in the Pole Vault at 14'6", this is before fiberglass poles I'd better tell you that; but anyway, like a flash of lightening it dawned on me—I can be an Olympic Champion.

I can't tell you what it is, this idea that you can do it, this faith, this something. I can tell you it gives meaning to every sprint down the runway, you work harder, you begin to lift weights, and you train like you've never trained before because you believe you can do it. Now I'm aware that there are 100,000 boys in America bigger than I am, stronger than I am, faster than I am, they could have beaten me; but I know that the determining factor is not so much ability but what you think you can do! I'm confident that I won a Gold Medal at the Olympics primarily because I believed I could win a Gold Medal at the Olympics. It's the greatest power in life."

But let's take a look at the above from a negative point of view. Who would have given a guy walking down the streets of Vienna, Austria a chance of taking over Germany? Here was this bedraggled guy, frustrated, deranged in mind, mad at everybody. In prison he wrote a book entitled "Mien Kampf—My Struggle". What he was going to do with the world, with the Jews. People laughed because they said, "This idiot will never take over Germany." Sixty million people lost their lives trying to stop that guy from accomplishing his ends. He believed he could do it, and while good people were standing by, Adolph Hitler took over the Third Reich. You can be what you want to be, it works for evil as well as good.

Think of a little pip-squeak of a guy, Lenin, walking into Moscow, Russia saying, "I'm going to take over Russia!" No one believed he could do it, but he did just that; and much of the chaos of the world today is because he accomplished his goal.

A man can be what he wants to be, and while good people are saying it can't be done, evil men are doing it—because they believe they can!

I think of one lone man who stood on the Grecian shore and said, "I'm going to win this world to Christ!" The Greeks said, "We'll out-think you, we'll out rationalize you, we'll out reason you." So this little guy stepped on the Roman shore and said, "I'm going to win this world to Christ!" The Romans laughed even harder. They said, "We'll squash you like one little thumbprint". And yet, 100 years later the Greco-Roman world was won to Christ because Paul believed that it could be done! The world belongs to the people of faith, to the people who believe they can do it. The future belongs to young men and women who will believe and will pay the price for making their dreams come true.

And lastly, DEDICATION is more important than ability. If you really want to be motivated, you've got to dedicate your life to something, commit yourself to something. I know we are prone to think that what really makes greatness in living is the man or woman with fantastic ability; a seven foot basketball player, a 300 pound lineman, that's what makes for greatness. The ability, the GOD-given inheritance. I don't deny that. I'm aware of the fact that ability is important. But more important than ability is the dedication of your life. The dedicated person will go beyond the person with ability alone.

When Peter Snell, the great runner, broke the mile World Record of 3:51.1 seconds everyone was amazed because the newspaper account said, "Peter Snell ran 15 miles home to tell his Mother about it." That shouldn't have shocked anyone because Peter Snell ran 20 miles per day. This fellow who held the mile record and also the half-mile record broke the half-mile record by 17 yards, not by a tenth of a second, not by a quarter of an inch, but by 17 yards. But do you want to know how he did it? Twenty miles per day! There are people reading this right now who could break the current world's record, but you know how you do it? Twenty-One miles per day!

Coaches talk about what makes a champion. Some say it's work. Others say no, it's a great coach; if a guy or girl has a great coach that coach will pull out their abilities. Some say no, it's the opportunity; given a certain set of circumstances any boy or girl, man or woman, would emerge great, it's the opportunity that makes the difference. Others say no, it's pure GOD-given natural ability that makes a champion. Still others say it's inspiration, the friendly word of encouragement.

Well, you and I know all of these things are important. But it is out of the burning desire to excel, out of the heart, to achieve a goal that a person does work. They will take coaching, they will beg for it! They will seize their opportunities, they will use their abilities to their utmost capacity, and they will drink inspiration. You show me a person with no desire, no goal and I can make a prediction. They will simply not work, they will not take coaching, opportunities will never be seized, and talents will lie unexpressed and undiscovered within them. Inspiration falls on them like water on a ducks back.

I believe the sports world lives with portraying one basic thing for living: The burning desire to succeed! This is why I think kids should play the games according to the rules of fair play. I think here is where kids can see it, they can see that out of ambition set on great goals and great concepts, out of events and athletes they might see in person, but these ambitions which can lift the mental horizon and can ultimately become a burning desire; out of that can come greatness in human life.

Records don't come easy; they are the products of fantastic dedication, thousands of hours of work. You can stretch your ability, you can stretch your mental capacity, you can stretch your physical capacity, and you can stretch every aspect of your being if you will dedicate and give your life to something great.

I close this chapter with this one last story—a story that took place many years ago in Moscow, Russia. The United States of America had come over there to meet the Russians in a dual track and field meet. Talk about a symbol of the world's struggle, here it was! Hardly a point was separating them. Athletes from these two great nations were battling right down to the wire, sprinting into the tape, jumping, throwing; competing for the glory of their nation.

Well, there were two boys battling for the High Jump Championship of the World. Here was John Thomas 6'5" tall and here was Valery Brumel at 6'1". Which one would you pick to jump 7'4 ½ inches in the air? The crossbar was set at a new World Record height. John Thomas tried his first jump and couldn't quite get over the bar. Valery Brumel went over the bar 3 inches, dropped on it, the crossbar shimmied off. John Thomas tried his second jump and still couldn't make it, the bar shimmied off. Valery Brumel went over the bar 4 inches, landed on top of the crossbar, it shimmied off. And then a torrential rain hit Moscow. Tons of water dropped onto the stadium; you couldn't even see across the stadium the rain was so heavy.

Thirty-five minutes later the television commentator said, "No one's going to jump in this because the take-off area is nothing but mud." But the judges decided that they had to go ahead and get the last jump, the final jump of the competition.

Sixty five thousand Russians poured back into the stadium. John Thomas tried his third jump, slipped in the mud, couldn't get over the bar; it was a good effort under the circumstances. They put the crossbar back up and 35 yards back you could see "fire" in Valery Brumel's eyes. Have you ever seen fire in a man's eyes? Dedication so determined that he's got to do it regardless of anything—there was fire in Valery Brumel's eyes! He sprinted like mad to his take-off mark, through the puddle, planted his take-off foot, and UGHH! He went over the crossbar 5 inches! You could hear the Russian crowd roar for the next 15 minutes YAHHH, YAHHH, YAHHH!

You want the story? When Valery Brumel was 12 years old he said, "I'm going to break the high jump record for the glory of my nation." Seven years later without being out of shape one day, at the age of 19 he broke the world's record. That's what I mean by dedication!

If you want the symbol of the problems of the world, I tell you that little high jump contest is a picture of the world. You know why the Russians have beaten us for so many years? They're dedicated! They are more dedicated to a wrong cause than we are to a right cause.

Dedication made America. This great nation is what it is because people sacrificed. There is more to life than a country club existence, four wheels and a good time. If we are going to go down in history as "The Greatest Nation" we are going to have to re-discover dedication. The dedicated nation rises while the non-dedicated nation goes down.

I think of Moscow stadium. There was a boy still down on the field doing push-ups. All the Russians had left; there was no one in the stadium. John Gudnik was out there doing push-ups; the Russian Bolotnikov had beaten him. As he was doing these push-ups, Bob Richards came up to him and said, "John, what are you doing?" He said, "I'm doing push-ups, Bob." Bob said, "I know, I can see that—but why?" John Gudnik looked up, sweating, salt running into his mouth, tired, worn-out and he said, "Bob, I was beaten today, I'm not going to be beaten the next time I meet Bolotnikov!"

You want the secret in space, you want the secret in the Olympics, you want to build a spiritual life, a community, a Nation, the Kingdom of GOD. Here it is friends—DEDICATION, DEDICATION!

CHAPTER TWO

TRAINING THE BODY FOR PEAK PERFORMANCE

TRAINING FOR PEAK PERFORMANCE

When I started my coaching career in 1962, I coached the way I was coached, ultimately following someone else's mistakes. Unfortunately, so did a lot of other coaches. Wrestling coaches, for example, allowed the very dangerous practice of dehydration weight loss. They enjoyed the flexibility of having a wrestler lose weight to wrestle in a lower weight class. Exercise, rubber suits, voluntary dehydration, and even diuretics and saunas were used (and unfortunately still are), to sweat off pounds to make weight. We now know that with as little as a 2% weight loss from dehydration, the athlete begins losing strength, which can lead to losing a match regardless of the coaches ranting and raving.

Some state high school associations have now adopted minimal wrestling weight regulations to avoid this practice. Things relative to these weight-loss practices began to change in 1997 when in a span of two months, three collegiate wrestlers died of heat stroke caused by dehydration weight loss.

The American College of Sports Medicine position stand on weight loss in wrestling is now calculated by using body composition techniques to determine fat-free weight and percent body fat. Wrestlers may not compete below a weight equal to fat-free weight plus 5% body fat measured in the hydrated state. This program eliminates the need for dehydration weight loss as well as the unhealthy "starve and stuff" practice once common to this sport. Hopefully, this practice will be implemented in all high schools in all states.

I was lucky enough, after 5 years of doing what all the other coaches were doing, to meet Dr. Barry S. Brown, Ph.D. in Exercise Physiology at the University of Arkansas (now retired), at a luncheon. They didn't have Exercise Physiology when I went to San Jose State University, and I was fascinated by what Dr. Brown was telling me when I asked about our training methods. I ultimately went to his university to learn all I could about training methods and energy systems. What a blessing this was to the advancement of my coaching career.

General Training Concepts

It is important to remember that everyone has enormous potential, but each of us will respond differently to that potential, especially to exercise. Interestingly enough, a positive response occurs only when the body is **ready** to respond. Physically immature individuals lack the physiological capability to respond completely to muscular or fitness training demands. As an example, pre-pubertal boys may gain some strength in a resistance training program, but will gain a lot more after puberty when the level of the growth hormone testosterone is elevated.

In addition, proper nutrition and rest are keys to benefiting from any training program. There is also psychological readiness, which refers to a level of maturity necessary for the individual to make the commitment and sacrifices necessary to achieve peak performance.

We all have a great capacity for improvement, but very few, including the athlete, come close to reaching that potential. Studies have shown that Olympic medals are correlated to a country's average daily caloric intake. You can't excel without the energy necessary to train or without good coaching, competition, and the will to sacrifice for success.

Athletes will also respond differently to the same training program. Heredity, maturity, diet, sleep, and other personal and environmental factors will also influence individual responses.

Principles of Training

The type of training you do must be related to whatever it is you want to accomplish. This principle applies to the muscles involved and to the energy systems within those muscles.

Example: when you run, you recruit certain muscle fibers, energy pathways, and energy sources. Running every day trains the muscle fibers used in running. The body will adapt to endurance training differently than it does to strength training. Cycling is not the best training for running and vice versa. Why? Because the two activities use different muscle fibers. Studies have shown that the best results always come with specific training. However, some cycling could be good for a runner in that it provides relief from the pounding of running, provides muscle balance and trains adjacent muscle fibers.

Moderation: Applies to all aspects of life. If you train too hard, too fast or too long, the body begins to deteriorate. Too much of anything can be bad for physical and psychological health.

Warm-up and Cool Down: Warming up will increase your body temperature, respiration and heart rate; and helps protect against muscle, tendon, and ligament strains. Be aware of the fact that flexibility or stretching is more effective after warm-up than before.

Cool-down is just as important as the warm-up because stopping a workout too soon can lead to pooling of the blood, sluggish circulation, and slow removal of waste products. Light activity and stretching continue the pumping action of muscles on veins, helping circulation in the removal of metabolic byproducts such s lactic acid. Cool-down can also contribute to less cramping, soreness, or more serious problems such as heart rhythm problems in older athletes.

Overload: Leads to changes in the muscles used in training, thus stimulating the production of new protein to help meet future exercise demands. These changes occur in the systems that support and supply the exercise. The nervous system learns to recruit muscle fibers more effectively and coordinating systems become better able to supply oxygen and fuel to the working muscles. Training **must** place a demand on the muscle if you want positive results. As the body adapts to increases in workload you must increase the size of the load. Improvement is directly related to Frequency, Intensity and Time (duration). **Frequency** is the number of sessions per day, week, month or year. **Intensity** is the training load per day, week, month or year. **Time** is the length of training in hours per day, week, month or year.

Adaptation: The best you can do is follow a sensible training program, keep good records and make adjustments when and where necessary. Training cannot be rushed. You can't accomplish all of your goals in one session; trying to do this can cause more harm than good.

Recovery: The importance of allowing time for recovery must not be ignored. Training should progress from general to specific, from part to whole, and quantity to quality.

Variation: Training must be varied to help eliminate boredom and to maintain interest. Bodily changes occur when overload is followed by rest, and hard training is followed by easy periods to allow for recovery.

Follow a long workout with a short one, or high speed with easy distance.

Periodization: Is a very common term used today. It is simply the process of dividing training into smaller and larger sections or cycles which helps ensure proper training stimulus and time for recovery. In strength training, this calls for periods of strength, power, and endurance with each period lasting from several weeks to months, and each is divided into smaller cycles allowing for increasing loads, rest and recovery.

Longevity: In sports like gymnastics, female athletes may reach elite status at a relatively young age, before maturity affects the ratio of strength to body weight. Other sports, where aerobic fitness and muscular fitness are paramount, athletes may have to train for years to reach their potential.

Regression: Most of the adaptations the body makes to training are reversible; they may be lost when training is stopped. It takes approximately 3 times as long to gain endurance as it does to lose it. With complete bed rest, aerobic fitness declines at a rate of 9% per week. Strength is lost at a slower rate, but lack of use weakens even the best-trained muscles and in time the muscle undergoes atrophy, or decrease in size.

This helps to explain why over-training is a very big risk. It can lead to illness or injury, and both can put a halt to training, which contributes to regression. This is also why off-season training is so important; so you don't lose hard earned gains made in training.

Facts & Myths in Training

"No Pain, No Gain"

*Training is often difficult and sometimes unpleasant, but it shouldn't hurt. Pain is **not** a natural result of training. During exercise the body produces natural opiates called endorphins that can mask (cover up) discomfort from the effort. If real pain is experienced, back off!*

Discomfort is fine and is a natural result of the hydrogen ion (acid) build that accompanies the anaerobic (without oxygen) effect of lifting weights or intervals, or of muscle fatigue, microscopic muscle damage, and soreness that comes with distance work.

Discomfort coming 24 hours after exercise is called "delayed onset muscle soreness." I'll talk about this later.

You Must Tear Down Muscle To Build Muscle – Go for the Burn!

Excessive trauma to the muscle will not improve training: it will actually stop it! Weightlifters can traumatize muscles by overworking them; lifting too much weight or doing too many repetitions. This is **NOT** a necessary part of developing strength. Neither pain or damaging a muscle should be part of training; you should avoid both.

Micro-trauma (cell damage) will occur in muscles during hard training and competition but it isn't necessary or even desirable. Marathon runners will sometimes exhibit micro-trauma at the end of a marathon; running downhill, which requires eccentric contractions (the muscle lengthens while contracting) will cause micro-trauma to the muscles involved. In fact, this has been shown to be a major cause of muscle soreness, often leading to several weeks of necessary recovery time.

The phrase "go for the burn" is often heard in the gym with weightlifters doing a lot of sets and/or repetitions to supposedly build, shape and define muscles. The "burn" they talk about is probably due to the increased acidity associated with elevated levels of lactic acid in the muscle. Though this feeling, or sensation, is not dangerous, it isn't a necessary part of a strength program supposedly designed to improve performance.

Lactic Acid Causes Muscle Soreness

This one has been around since before I started coaching in 1962 and has absolutely no basis in fact. It's true that lactic acid is produced during muscle contractions that result in soreness, but the lactic acid isn't the direct causes of the soreness. Why? Because lactic acid is cleared from the muscle and blood within an hour after you stop exercising, while soreness peaks 24 to 48 hours later—long after the lactic acid is removed or metabolized.

Delayed onset muscle soreness, referred to above in "No Pain, No Gain" will follow any exercise your body (muscles) are not familiar with, vigorous effort after a long layoff or eccentric (lengthening) muscle contractions. This delayed soreness is associated with micro-trauma to the muscle and connective tissue, swelling or fluid build-up (edema), and leakage of substances from the muscle (e.g., the enzyme creatine kinase).

After a long recovery period, often days or weeks, the athlete basically becomes immune to further soreness from this particular exercise or movement; but only from this particular activity (the one that caused the initial soreness).

Muscle Can Turn To Fat or Vice Versa

When you stop training, does your muscle turn to fat? **NO!** Both muscle and fat are very specialized tissues, each with a very specific purpose.

Muscle fibers are composed of long, thin strands of contractile protein specifically designed to exert force. Training will increase the size of muscle fiber (hypertrophy), and stopping training (detraining) will reduce their size (atrophy). When you stop training, some fat can be deposited among the fibers if energy intake is greater than energy output; but long, thin muscle fibers do **NOT** change into fat cells.

Fat cells are spherical blobs designed to store fat. They grow in size when you store fat and shrink when you lose weight. These globular fat cells can **NOT** take on the duties of muscle fibers.

There is something called intramuscular fat, a small amount of fat that can be stored in endurance trained muscle fibers, but this is less than 0.1% of the body's total. This is the first fat oxidized during exercise. If the effort continues, additional fat will be used from adipose tissue deposits (usually subcutaneous abdominal) and will be transported to the muscle through the circulatory system (blood).

I "Ran Out of Wind"

If you are asking your body to perform at a level beyond your conditioning level, you will experience the feeling of running out of air, or wind. This sensation comes from the lungs and is most likely due to excess carbon dioxide (CO_2) rather than to a lack of oxygen. Carbon dioxide is produced during the oxidative metabolism of carbohydrate, and CO_2 is the primary stimulus that drives respiration.

When CO_2 levels are high, as in vigorous exercise, it causes distress signals as the lungs attempt to blow off the excess. As a result, the respiratory system thinks it is more important to rid the body of excess CO_2 than it is to bring in more oxygen.

Having too much CO_2 is a sign that you have gone past your lactate threshold and that you are working above the level you trained for. You should become familiar with this sensation and what it means; if you ignore it during training or competition you will become exhausted.

Nutrition and Rest

If you fail to eat properly and lack the energy to train properly, the essential amino acids, vitamins, and minerals needed to support muscle growth and the requirements of training will not be available to respond properly to the demands being placed on your body. Training requires enough protein to build muscle enzymes, and other structures influenced by training and to repair muscle damaged in vigorous effort.

- A **non-athlete** needs about **0.8 grams** of protein per 2.2 pounds (1 kilogram) of body weight per day.

- An **endurance athlete** requires about **1.2 – 1.4 grams** of protein per 2.2 pounds (1 kilogram) of body weight per day.

- A **strength athlete** may need **1.4 – 1.8 grams** of protein per 2.2 pounds (1 kilogram) of body weight per day.

Note: There are 25 grams of protein in a serving of beef about the size of a deck of cards (3 oz.).

As an example, basketball is a high-energy sport and practices can cause an athlete to burn 500-600 kilocalories per hour. This means the diet also needs adequate carbohydrate and sufficient fat to fuel the body. Too little carbohydrate, and the body will turn to protein to provide energy. Nutritious, complex carbohydrates, including fruits, vegetables beans, corn, rice, potatoes and whole-grain breads and pasta should constitute at least 60% of the athlete's diet to promote energy and conserve protein.

To get the winning edge, the athlete must fuel the body correctly. As Napoleon Bonaparte said, "An army marches on its stomach."

Growing athletes need a lot of rest. Most positive training adaptations occur during sleep; and sleep is vital to good health as well as performance. Adults who get 7-8 hours of sleep are healthier than those who get less than 7 or more than 9 hours of sleep.

How Do Muscles Work?

Muscles work by shortening when they are stimulated by the nervous system. Each muscle is surrounded by connective tissue, and so are the individual fibers within the muscle. All of these layers of connective tissue are continuous with tendons and fibrous sheaths that connect muscle to bone.

Muscle contractions are controlled by the brain via signals transported by nerves. Nerve impulses tell the muscle which fibers to contract, when to contract, and how long to maintain the contraction. The nervous system also coordinates multiple muscle contractions to cause smooth movements.

A muscle works by shortening when called upon by the nervous system. Connective tissue surrounds each muscle, as well as the individual fibers and small groups of fibers within each muscle. All of this connective tissue is continuous with tendons and fibrous sheaths that attach to the bones.

As a muscle contracts, the muscle fiber pulls the connective tissue that then pulls the tendons attached to the bone. Think of a muscle as a spring that can only pull—it cannot push! As a result, when muscles contract, they pull equally on the tendons attached to both ends of the muscle.

As an athlete learns a new skill they have to consciously think about what is happening in order to control the movement. This often results in poor coordination; but as the skill is practiced the resulting coordination becomes controlled.

Inside a Muscle (truly amazing):

Every skeletal muscle contains cells (fibers), connective tissue, blood vessels, nerves, and intramuscular fat. Each muscle cell also contains thousands of spaghetti-like fibers that extend along most of, if not the entire length, of the muscle. Within these fibers are thread-like strands called myofibrils which contain bundles of protein that slide over one another to cause muscle shortening (contraction) when stimulated by the nervous system, or relaxation when the stimulation stops. This is called the "sliding filament theory." If enough of the muscle fibers are stimulated, the muscle will shorten and the attached bone will move.

Each muscle has many slender nerve fibers that enter the body of the muscle. Each nerve splits when it enters the muscle and activates a set number of muscle fibers. The average nerve in skeletal muscle activates about 150 muscle fibers, called motor units.

The force of a given contraction depends on the number of motor units that are activated and the size of the motor unit. The force generated will be the result of the frequency of activation and number of motor units within a muscle that are stimulated.

There are very distinct differences among motor units that relate directly to the type of muscle fiber being recruited. These fibers can be distinguished as slow-oxidative (SO), fast oxidative-glycolytic (FOG), or fast-glycolytic (FG) fibers. Every muscle has a combination of SO, FOG, and FG motor units, the percentage of which varies according to muscle function, training, and genetics.

Slow-oxidative fibers contract slowly and are ideally suited for endurance work due to their high aerobic capacity (ability to use oxygen). FOG fibers share some of the characteristics of both SO and FG fibers that have been aerobically trained. FO fibers are more suited for short-term, intense anaerobic work (without oxygen).

The nervous system basically recruits SO fibers first, then adds additional fibers as more force and speed is needed.

Since muscles can only pull, muscles come in groups, with groups of muscles working together to allow movement in multiple directions. In addition to all of this, the shape and form of the muscle, along with fiber characteristics, determine the speed, force, and endurance of a specific movement.

Generally speaking, the attachment of muscle to bones is such that a slight shortening within a muscle can cause a large movement at the end of a limb (leverage). This allows us to generate high speeds of limb movement when it is needed.

While each person inherits a certain percentage of SO, FOG and FG muscle fibers, the way these fibers are used on a regular daily basis also influences the percentage of each fiber type. Research indicates that elite distance runners have a higher percentage of SO fibers while sprinters, high jumpers, etc. have more FG fibers.

The ability we have to move is truly AMAZING!

Muscle Soreness

It is important to understand that imperfect training can result in bad habits, so learning new skills properly is very important. There are basically two types of soreness associated with exercise training: short term and long term.

Short term may occur during or shortly after intense or extended exercise. This temporary soreness is probably due to acid-base imbalances, slight swelling, and the buildup of metabolic waste. These are all relieved within a short period of time.

Long term soreness that occurs the next day or lasts for several days is often due to the muscle lengthening (eccentric contractions) done during the exercise (as in running downhill). This residual pain, which begins 12-24 hours after exercise and can last up to two weeks, is called "delayed onset" muscle soreness. This delayed onset soreness can be avoided or minimized if training intensity is increased slowly, especially early in the season. The best idea is to avoid excess activities such as running downhill that cause the muscle to lengthen during contractions.

TRAINING THE RIGHT ENERGY SYSTEMS

The object here is to give you a positive approach to training the athlete. Knowing something about energy systems, what they do and how they work can really help the coach and athlete in designing a specific training program for a specific sport.

Our body must be continuously supplied with chemical energy in order to perform its many complex functions. Physical activity by far provides the greatest demand for energy. The energy output from working muscles may be 120 times higher than at rest. During less intense but sustained exercise such as cross country or marathon running the energy requirements increase 20-30 times above resting levels.

The body cannot maintain maximum, all out speed for longer than 6-10 seconds. As a result, additional energy must be generated for replenishment. Thus stored carbohydrates, fats and proteins stand ready to continuously recharge the body's stores for energy.

The energy in food is not transferred directly to the cells for biologic work (referred to as a "high energy phosphate"). This nutrient energy is funneled through the energy-rich compound Adenosine Triphosphate (ATP). About 40% of the potential energy in food is transferred to ATP. Creatine Phosphate (CP) serves as an energy reserve to rapidly replenish ATP when called upon.

Performance of short duration, high intensity exercises such as the 100 yard dash, 25 yard swim, sprinting in basketball, football, or soccer, require an immediate supply of energy. This energy comes almost exclusively from ATP and CP stored within the specific muscles being used.

All sports require utilization of high-energy phosphates, but many will rely on them exclusively. For example, success in football, basketball, track and field, weight lifting, baseball, volleyball, ice hockey, field hockey, wrestling, gymnastics, all will undoubtedly require a brief maximal effort during performance.

For sustained exercise and recovery from all-out effort, additional energy must be generated from stored carbohydrates, fats, and proteins in order to replenish ATP.

By understanding energy systems as well as the different types of muscle fibers (fast twitch and slow twitch), it is possible to train for specific improvement and help the athlete reach his or her "Peak Performance" level. But first, we need to define some terms we will be referring to in our discussion.

ATP (Adenosine Triphosphate) - is used for all cellular processes requiring energy. There is only a very small amount of ATP in the cell; the total quantity within the body at any one time is about 3 ounces (85 grams). This is why it is available to perform maximum exercise for only a few seconds.

Creatine Phosphate (CP) - is another high-energy phosphate. The cell's concentration of CP is about 3-5 times greater than ATP and is thus considered the high-energy reservoir.

Carbohydrates - supply energy for cellular work. It is the only nutrient whose stored energy can be used to generate ATP anaerobically (without oxygen); this is very important during vigorous high intensity exercise. A certain level of carbohydrate breakdown is required for fats to be metabolized; so to this extent fats burn in a carbohydrate flame.

Lactic Acid - should not be viewed as a metabolic "waste" product. It is a very valuable source of chemical energy that accumulates and is retained in the body during intense physical exercise. It is converted to pyruvic acid and is used as an energy source. The most rapidly accumulated and highest lactic acid levels are reached during exercise that can be sustained for 60-180 seconds. As the intensity of "all-out" exercise decreases, thereby extending the work period, there is a corresponding decrease in both the rate of build-up and the final level of lactic acid in the bloodstream. When untrained, healthy subjects reach about 55% of maximal capacity, lactic acid begins to accumulate. This lactic acid threshold increases with training.

Combination of Systems - Energy for exercise is not just the result of a series of energy systems that switch on and off, but rather the smooth blending with considerable overlap from one mode of energy transfer to another. For intense exercise of longer duration (1-2 minutes), energy is generated mainly from anaerobic reactions of glycolysis—a short-term energy system. As exercise progresses beyond several minutes, the aerobic system predominates and oxygen consumption becomes an important factor—a long-term energy system.

     The body can produce energy with oxygen (aerobically) or without it (anaerobically). Energy from anaerobic metabolism is produced by ATP (adenosine triphosphate) breaking down to adenosine disphosphate (ADP). ATP is the ultimate fuel all cells need. The energy to reconvert this ADP back to ATP is provided by creatine phosphate (CP) or phosphocreatine (PC).

     During vigorous exercise, when the lungs and bloodstream are not able to supply the oxygen demands of the muscles, lactic acid develops which builds up in the muscle and overflows into the bloodstream. A great deal of the lactic acid is transported by the liver, where it is reconverted into glycogen (muscle sugar). But a certain amount of lactic acid builds up in the muscle and can contribute to premature muscle exhaustion, the typical burning sensation.

     During intense exercise, exhaustion coincides with depletion of muscle glycogen (sugar). So what happens if ATP, PC and glycogen are all depleted? An energy source kicks in from the metabolism of carbohydrates (glucose) and fats. In this case, fat is a rather poor source of energy because it metabolizes slowly. It gets better with intensive training which means you can delay glycogen depletion by burning fat instead; a tune-up job (getting into good physical condition). This is called "glycogen sparing". Glycogen stores are increased when a high carbohydrate diet is used.

It is interesting to note here that fat people have more trouble burning up fat than lean people; muscle burns calories and most fat people don't have enough of it.

Many athletes involved in high-intensity sports do not focus enough on consuming a high carbohydrate training diet or carbohydrates just prior to their event because it hasn't been traditionally believed to be critical to their performance. Research now almost uniformly has shown that a low-carbohydrate diet (3-15% carbohydrate) impairs performance of high intensity single or multiple sets compared to a moderate or high carbohydrate intake. Since there is no known detriment to consumption of a high carbohydrate diet, other than weight gain due to water retention, it is recommended that all athletes consume a high carbohydrate training diet, i.e., at least 70% of energy as carbohydrate (7-10 grams per kilogram of weight), and increase this to 85% for the few days before competition. Use of a carbohydrate supplement (see Chapters Three and Four for recommendations) before and during exercise will likely improve performance of intermittent, high-intensity work.

What Happens Inside a Muscle During Exercise?

Let's use a run as an example. As the run starts, muscle fiber gets energy from two stored compounds, ATP (adenosine triphosphate) and PC (phosphocreatine). Since these two energy sources are in short supply, the muscle will run out of energy after about 10 seconds; but just as the ATP and PC are running low the muscle starts to use stored carbohydrate (glycogen) to produce more ATP. As glycogen begins to breakdown, lactic acid begins to appear in the muscle and acid by-products can reduce energy and the ability to produce force. As a result, another energy source has to step up or fatigue will result. So after a couple of minutes the muscle gets its "second wind" as the cardio-respiratory system provides more oxygen for the formation of more

ATP, which comes from the breakdown (oxidation) of carbohydrates and fat. When the runner begins to increase the pace, the muscle will recruit fast-twitch fibers that depend on muscle glycogen to produce ATP. Unfortunately, the amount of muscle glycogen is also limited and won't last more than 1 or 2 hours. As a result, another energy source, blood glucose, supplied from glycogen stored in the liver, is called into action. Finally, when muscle and liver glycogen have run out, the muscle is forced to rely on fat for energy. This is when the runner begins to slow down, because the ability of the body to utilize energy (energy metabolism) is not as efficient when it runs out of carbohydrate, since more oxygen is required to burn fat. This is exactly why a diet high in carbohydrates is so vitally important!

Energy Systems

The energy for muscle contraction comes from two energy systems, the anaerobic (without oxygen) and aerobic (with oxygen) systems.

The Anaerobic System

Since the supply of stored compounds necessary to produce "non-oxidative" (without oxygen) energy is so limited, anaerobic effort is brief (10 seconds or less) but intense. This energy system is critical for events of short duration and also fuels the sprint or kick at the end of a longer event. In running events like 400 to 800 meters, the goal is to run out of anaerobic energy as the finish line is crossed. In events of longer duration and sports with continuous motion, like soccer, basketball, and rugby, the athlete alternates between anaerobic and aerobic energy systems. Thus, one of the great benefits of aerobic fitness is that it improves the ability to recover from anaerobic bursts of effort, such as a fast break in basketball.

The Aerobic System

These energy pathways use large amounts of carbohydrate and fat to provide ATP for muscle contraction. Muscle that has been trained for endurance contains more fat, and highly trained endurance muscles have the ability to efficiently use fat for energy, even during moderately intense activity. A large aerobic capacity, ability to utilize oxygen, is critical for performance in all sports. This makes an off-season long distance training program extremely valuable for any sport, because you can significantly increase your VO_2 Maximum (volume of oxygen capacity.

Aerobic capacity, (VO_2 Max), is an excellent predictor of performance in non-weight bearing sports such as cycling, swimming, and rowing. It is also a predictor of performance in weight-bearing activity such as running, cross-country skiing, and speed skating. Basically, a high aerobic capacity can have a positive effect on performance in all sports. If you can have a VO_2 Max test done can be a great motivator as you see your aerobic capacity numbers improve during training.

Aerobic metabolism is the most efficient pathway of energy production. What happens during endurance exercise? During the first 5-10 minutes of a long distance run, muscle glycogen (muscle sugar - carbohydrate) is the major fuel consumed. After 10-40 minutes the muscle uses glucose from the bloodstream. After 60-240 minutes of exercise, the working muscle begins to oxidize fatty acid. This increased fatty acid usage in the physically fit person seems to decrease glucose uptake and may help in preventing hypoglycemia (low-blood sugar), during extended exercise.

The intensity of exercise also plays a part in determining the fuel used for energy production. At "moderate" levels of exercise, energy production is about 50% from fat and 50% from carbohydrate. As exercise intensity increases, the body tends to rely on carbohydrate rather than fat, and this can cause problems since fat stores are much more plentiful than carbohydrate stores. The untrained person will quickly elevate the heart-rate and approach his or her maximum tolerance for work, relying on limited stores of carbohydrate, while the well-trained person does the same amount of work with a lower heart-rate and at less than maximum tolerance and can continue to use more plentiful fatty acid, which yields more energy per gram than does carbohydrate.

Late stages of prolonged exercise often lead to an inability of the body to maintain blood glucose (sugar) which may be an important sign of impending fatigue. Carbohydrate feeding during exercise can help delay this onset of fatigue. Every 15-20 minutes during prolonged exercise, athletes should drink 8-12 ounces of a sports drink containing carbohydrate (not one high in simple sugar and sodium), or fruit juice to replace carbohydrate and fluid. This will prevent a fall in blood glucose and will likely delay fatigue.

Muscle Fiber Types

A great deal has been written about muscle fiber types in various athletes. Endurance athletes, such as long distance runners, have more red (slow twitch) muscle fibers than white (fast twitch) fibers, which are common in athletes participating in anaerobic (without oxygen) activities such as weightlifting, sprinting, and football. Since white fibers cannot be changed into red fibers with training, or visa versa it is important for the athlete to get maximum performance out of the various muscle types he or she has.

A rather simple method for finding out which athletes in your group have which type of fiber is to have each athlete stand with their side against a wall; have them reach as high as possible and make a mark with a piece of chalk. Now have them jump from a standing position, off both feet, as high as possible and make a second mark. Measure the difference between mark one and mark two. The athlete with the greatest distance between the two marks has the greatest amount of fast twitch (white) muscle fiber in their calves; therefore having the most potential for speed and quickness. Athletes having the lowest measurement from first to second mark are the ones with more (slow twitch) muscle fiber; therefore possibly being you slowest runners and possibly the best long distance athletes. Those with the intermediate scores, based upon analysis of your particular group, have a balance of fast and slow twitch muscle fibers and are potentially middle distance runners in track or positions not requiring as much speed and quickness as in other sports.

What Are You Training For?

I get very concerned as I travel worldwide watching athletes train, coaches train the athletes, and athletes perform trying to figure why they are doing what they are doing. I can remember back to when I was playing sports in high school and college not really knowing what I was doing during training and why we were doing various drills and exercises. When I started my coaching career I was told to do certain drills and exercises with the athletes, not really understanding why.

Fortunately I had the opportunity to meet Dr. Barry S. Brown, Ph.D. from the University of Arkansas, one of the finest exercise physiologists in the world. I began asking questions about training techniques and energy systems, and found out there was a whole new world out there in exercise physiology that could lead to peak performance. I started asking questions and Dr. Brown started giving me answers that have changed my entire approach to coaching and teaching.

The question I want to ask each of you is WHY? I want parents to understand why the athletes are doing what they are doing, I want the coaches to understand what they are making the kids do and why they are doing it, and I want the athletes to understand what they are being asked to do.

Remember this in weight training? Do three sets of 10! Why?

Why not do one set of 30 and go home? Are you training adenosine triphosphate, phosphocreatine, lactic acid, glycogen or fat? Are you training a fast twitch or slow twitch muscle fiber? Are you training for strength, power, quickness or endurance or some combination? If you don't know which of these you are training for and why, how can you expect to receive maximum benefit from the training program? The answer is, you can't! So let's talk about getting maximum performance training the body inside out.

Training Energy Systems

I want you to snap your fingers! In order to do this there is a little chemical in each muscle cell we have referred to already called ATP (adenosine triphosphate). It is a chemical that makes the muscle (cell) move. This system, the ATP/PC system allows the muscle to perform maximally for 6-10 seconds; it is a no-oxygen or anaerobic system. The longest amount of time a muscle can perform wide open all-out is 10 seconds. It is not physiologically possible to ask an athlete to do anything wide open for longer than 10 seconds because you run out of this ATP.

How many of you remember running wind sprints when you were in school? We would, during football and basketball, run up and down the field or gym floor as fast as we could. Coaches wanted us to run wide open from one end to the other, then turn around and do it again, and again, and again. They wanted the 2nd, 3rd and 4th, sprint to be just as fast as the first one. Finally we were bent over, gasping for air until finally someone got sick and threw up.

Our coaches thought this was wonderful. If you got sick you were really working hard. We got so good at this that we threw-up before practice because we knew what was going to happen during practice. What happened? We ran until we literally couldn't run anymore but never got in shape for the game of football. We always ran out of gas before the game ended. Fortunately most of our opponents got tired before we did.

Our coaches didn't understand which energy system we were training and how to make it perform optimally. In today's school systems and youth programs the coaches oftentimes are untrained in exercise physiology and many times are doing more harm to the athlete than good. At the end of 6-10 seconds of wide-open activity you run out of ATP and start going slower; no matter how many names you are being called or how hard you may try.

How long, for example, does a football play last? Ten seconds is about the longest any play will last; in fact the average is about 6 seconds. So it would seem logical to me that if I was going to train an athlete for football I would want to train the correct energy system (ATP/PC) and not the aerobic system once we start football practice in the fall. Any aerobic work should have been done during the off-season because football doesn't use this system. This ATP/PC ten second system is the only one he needs.

We will talk about other sports later, but you can begin thinking about any given sport and which energy system it requires. For now let's concentrate on football. Here is what I would do when the team gathers for the first workout: I want you, the athlete, to start on this line; when I say "go" I want you to run all-out for 10 seconds or until you hear the whistle blow. When the whistle blows your distance from the starting point will be marked. Once you hear the whistle I want you to slow down and jog or walk for the next two minutes or until you recover and can talk normally again without huffing and puffing.

It must be understood that each athlete, regardless of the sport, is different here. Some need a longer recover time than others based upon their size and conditioning level when training begins. Make sure the athlete receives some water after each bout of exercise. Then the next 10-second sprint is performed.

Two or 3 days later the recovery period is cut to a minute and 45 seconds; two days later a minute and 30 seconds; two days later a minute and 15 seconds; two days later one minute, and so on. At the end of 2-3 weeks of training the young person can run wide open for 10 seconds during a game. By the time he gets out from underneath the pile, gets back to the huddle, defense or offense, gets the next play and walks back up to the line of scrimmage all of the ATP has been recovered and he can perform maximally. I can now tell the athletes there is no excuse for getting tired during a game because we have trained the correct energy system for maximum performance, and the athlete can understand this.

Football coaches will often say, "You know why we lost the game? Our defense was on the field the whole game and simply got tired?" Why? Weren't you playing against someone? How come your team got tired and they didn't? You should be able to recover adequately between plays. It is a matter of training the correct energy system in order to give you maximum performance capability.

Now, if we continue to run the athlete, wide-open, for longer than 10 seconds he or she will begin to slow down. They have to because they ran out of ATP. The body now switches to another energy system called the "lactate" system, which is still an "anaerobic" no oxygen system. How many of you have ever walked up hill, rode a bicycle, walked up steps and got a little "burn" in your legs?

This is lactic acid and if it builds up too much you can't perform because of muscle fatigue. However, this system is used for energy while your ATP/PC system is recovering and allows you to perform at the next level of intensity, a lower speed, from about 10 seconds to about 3 minutes. In track and field this would be somewhere between 200 to 800 meters. But it is still a system that is not using oxygen for energy. You are using almost all carbohydrates; muscle sugar.

Now I ask the athlete to keep running as fast as possible. But he or she can't keep the initial or secondary speed up so they begin to slow down some more. The body switches energy gears again and now goes to the glycogen system or aerobic system (with oxygen). You are running slower but much more efficiently. This system runs primarily from 2-3 minutes to two hours as your primary source of energy.

Finally, about the two-hour mark you begin to burn fat as your primary source of energy.

As a coach working with long distance athletes I am going to spend most of my time working on this "fat burning" system; running longer and slower so the body learns how to use fat as its primary fuel. It doesn't mean that I don't do speed work with the athlete, it means that the emphasis is on training the energy system that is used most during this particular sport or event within a sport.

What about other sports like soccer? Which energy systems are at work here? Probably 2 of the four (ATP/PC, and blood lactate) meaning the athlete has to do sprint work, plus intermediate sprints during training. Basketball and ice hockey would be the same. Baseball uses only one energy system, ATP/PC. Swimming and track, depending upon the event, might use all four energy systems: ATP/PC, lactate, glycogen and FAT. The point here is that if you are using long distance work to train a sprinter during the season, you are defeating the purpose of your training. Energy systems are very sports-specific.

During the off season in most sports, some long distance training can be beneficial in building up the athletes VO_2 max, or maximum oxygen uptake. Let me give you an example here: Take a big breath! Now exhale! The actual amount of oxygen you delivered to the working muscle can be measured in milliliters of oxygen per kilogram of body weight per minute and is called your VO_2 max.

Long distance training has the effect of elevating this number. The higher the number, out of a maximum possible score of 100, the more oxygen you are able to deliver to the working muscle during a given activity. The more oxygen you can deliver to the working muscle the better the performance capability of the muscles being used.

So the baseball, soccer, basketball, football, ice hockey, or volleyball player can do long distance training off-season to help increase this oxygen delivery system which in turn can aid them during their actual sport. However, once the actual training season begins, 3-4 weeks prior to the first competition, the actual energy system(s) being used must be trained specifically. Once the athlete understands what they are being asked to do and why they are doing it, it is easier to get 100% effort from the athlete during training.

Make sure that athletes during training are allowed to get plenty of good cold water. Once the athlete starts to dehydrate you immediately lose performance and create all kinds of health risks. Remember, 78% of a muscle is water, all of the blood is water and up to 70% of your body is water. No water = no performance!

I have personally spent over 30 years coaching both football and gymnastics. Over this time period I have never lost a game or a match. I've been beat many times! You're going to have to beat me; you're going to have to have better athletes than me. But I know one thing for sure: we are not going to get tired during the game or competition! This simply means that I can walk up to any of my athletes after a workout or game and say, "Did you give me everything you had while you were out there?"

If I hear, "Yes sir!" I can say, "Good job!" He or she gave me everything they had, what more can I expect? In my personal opinion this is WINNING and what WINNING is all about! But the athlete should also expect that I gave everything I had, too. The coach owes it to the athlete to know which energy system does what and how to train the athlete properly so maximum performance can be expected. The coach, in my opinion, also owes it to the parent, to let them know what the athletes are being asked to do and why. Many times I have heard parents ask an athlete, "What did you do today?" The answer is, "We ran wind sprints until we got sick, did this, this and this!" The parent says, "Why?" and athlete responds with, "I don't know, we just did what we were told." Well, I think you had better know!

So in quick review:

the ATP/PC energy system lasts from 1-10 seconds
the Blood Lactate system from 10 seconds to 2-3 minutes
the Glycogen system from 2-3 minutes to 2 hours
then the Fat system takes over

Obviously there are some overlaps between the systems, which is exactly why training sometimes includes more than one.

ACHIEVING "TOTAL FITNESS"

Though it is difficult to precisely define "fitness", "total fitness" requires adequate muscular strength and endurance, reasonable joint flexibility, an efficient cardiovascular system with a good level of aerobic fitness, and acceptable body composition with control over body weight.

Principles of Conditioning:

Overload - Exercising the body at a level above that which it normally operates. This principle can be accomplished by increasing the frequency of exercise, increasing the intensity of exercise, or increasing the duration of exercise.

Specificity: This refers to the metabolic and physiologic changes that occur depending upon the type of overload used. Research studies suggest that a person should perform training exercises in a manner as close as possible to the way he or she wishes to use the improved capacity. Example: fitness for bicycling is best achieved through cycling exercises, and so on for other sports or activities.

Individual Difference - It is critical that the person's relative fitness level at the start of training is considered prior to prescribing an exercise program. Training benefits are maximized when programs are planned to meet individual needs and capabilities.

Reversibility - The "if you don't use it you lose it" principle. Once an individual reaches a certain level of conditioning, a regular program of activity must be maintained to prevent deconditioning. Some researchers have estimated that improvements gained are lost in 5-10 weeks, and often times much faster, once the conditioning is stopped.

Conditioning the Muscles of the Body

The overload principle is applied by the use of weights, immovable bars, straps, pulleys, or springs. The muscle will respond to the intensity of overload. The overload is created by increasing the load or resistance, the repetitions performed, the speed of muscular contraction, or by various combinations. Three systems are commonly used: Isotonic training, Isometric training and Isokinetic training.

Isotonic training, often referred to as weight training, involves the muscle exerting tension in order to overcome a fixed or variable resistance. There are two types of muscular contractions: Eccentric, the muscle lengthens as it contracts, and Concentric, the muscle shortens as it contracts.

Isometric training has no movement during the muscle contraction. One disadvantage to this method is that strength development is specific to the angle at which the force is applied. Another is that there is little if any transfer of isometric strength developed at one joint angle to other body positions, even when the same muscles are involved.

Isokinetic training is working against a resistance that permits movement at a pre-set, pre-fixed speed and enables the muscle to obtain its maximum contraction throughout the full range of movement.

Don't plan on using weight training as your primary source of aerobic training. A one-hour weight training session is usually no longer than about 6-8 minutes of actual muscular work.

Selecting Your Training Program

The following items must be considered prior to beginning your program:

- What are your personal objectives? Power training (strength vs. time) is usually six repetitions or less; strength training 7-15 repetitions; strength with muscle endurance 15-25 repetitions; muscle endurance training only 25-50 repetitions.

- How to get the most use of the available facilities and/or equipment. What is best for you relative to time, convenience and motivation factors?

- Selection of proper exercises.

- Proper arrangement of the exercises.

Anaerobic Conditioning

The capacity to perform all out exercise of up to 120 seconds in duration depends mainly on this system of energy metabolism. The overload system must be applied in conditioning in order to improve this energy generating capacity. Sports such as football, ice hockey and weightlifting rely mostly on energy derived from the anaerobic system and basically do not require oxygen. Thus a subsequent exercise bout can begin only after an adequate rest period for recovery. Individuals should undertake numerous bouts of intense, short duration exercise and the training activities selected must use the muscles for which the person desires anaerobic power.

Aerobic Conditioning

Continuous exercise performed for longer than two minutes requires energy from both the anaerobic and aerobic metabolic reactions. If the supply of oxygen is adequate to meet energy needs, then the exercise can be continued in a steady state and the feelings of discomfort from fatigue are minimal. Therefore the intensity at which exercise can be sustained for relatively long periods of time depends upon the body's capacity of support systems for oxygen transport, the heart, lungs and vascular system.

Before engaging in an aerobic exercise program you should consider the following factors:

Initial level of **cardiovascular capacity**.

Frequency of training. Three days per week minimum is generally accepted, although some adaptive changes may occur in two days per week.

Duration of training - continuous as well as intermittent overloads are effective in improving aerobic capacity. Even single 3-5 minute bouts of vigorous exercise performed 3 times per week will improve the aerobic system. Performing less exhausting but steady state exercise for 20 minutes or longer will increase the pumping ability of the heart and the metabolic capacity of the specific muscles used.

Intensity of training - this is a critical factor. The American College of Sports Medicine recommends that aerobic training, to be most efficient, be conducted 3 days per week utilizing 20-30 minutes of continuous exercise sufficient to expend about 300 kcal. This is usually assured by exercising at a pulse rate of about 70% of maximum heart rate (220 minus your age X 70%).

Specificity of Training - it is reasonable to advise that in training the aerobic system for a specific activity such as rowing, swimming, cycling, or running, the method of training must overload the appropriate muscles required by the activity as well as provide stress for the heart and vascular system.

Muscle Fiber Type - the average percentage of slow-twitch fibers in sedentary men is about 45-50 percent, but the variation is large. It would seem logical that these people, with a large proportion of slow twitch fibers in their leg muscles, would be successful in endurance running, while those with a distribution favoring fast twitch fibers would excel in sprint activities. It appears that the distribution of these fibers is determined by genetic code largely fixed at birth.

Start slowly, warm-up before you start any exercise program, dress sensibly, and allow a cool-down period of 5-10 minutes.

Training Muscles

Gains in strength are specific to the type of training being done. Therefore, a training program for a specific sport should consist predominantly of the types of muscular contraction encountered in that sport. It is relatively easy to design a training program for an individual but the coach's biggest challenge is to allow for individual responses to that program.

Need Analysis:

You should consider the following when designing a resistive exercise program:

- What muscle groups need to be trained?

- What are the basic energy sources (e.g. anaerobic, aerobic) that need to be trained?

- What type of muscle action (e.g. isometric, variable resistance) should be used?

- What are the primary sites of injury for the particular sport?

I want you to understand these terms:

Strength

When someone talks to you about "strength", what are they saying? Strength is the ability of a muscle to produce force. Strength, as defined by most exercise physiologists, is the maximal force you can exert in one voluntary muscle contraction. In other words, you might put an athlete on a bench and see how much weight they can bench-press one time. This is their strength factor.

All activity requires a certain amount of strength, but strength becomes a priority in sports where moving your body weight, lifting, carrying, or throwing or an object are involved.

The strength of a muscle corresponds directly to its cross-sectional size (how big it is). If resistance training is done properly, the number of fibers recruited for work can be increased. This is done by increasing contractile protein which increases contractile strength.

Strength is NOT related to muscle fiber type. Muscle fiber types, SO, FOG and FG, are all equal in strength when equal cross-sectional areas are compared. The difference is the speed at which they will generate force.

Power

Power is defined as work divided by time (or strength multiplied by velocity). The athlete who can do more work in the same amount of time has more power. What sports involve the use of power? Certainly most sports at one time or another use power.

The football player who can accelerate faster will reach the greatest velocity before a collision. In order to be more powerful, an athlete must be strong enough, regardless of the sport, to generate the necessary power. This is why a smaller defensive lineman in football may be able to outplay a larger offensive lineman. One athlete may have more strength, but the strength may not do any good if it can't be used properly.

For example, one football player can bench press 400 pounds, and another player only 300 pounds. Does this make the stronger player better? Of course not! It only means he can lift more weight one time. The player who actually lifts less weight, but can do it more often over a given time, may have a distinct advantage.

Muscular Endurance

Muscular endurance is the ability of a muscle to produce force repeatedly over a period of time, and usually involves small versus large muscle groups. It is measured by the number of repetitions which can be done at any one time.

Think of a sport in which you may need some muscle endurance, the ability to do muscular work more than just one time. Wouldn't it be nice to go to the ski hill during the winter and ski down the hill more than once? One person may be able to leg press 700 pounds once or twice in a row while another person (same age, height, and weight) can only leg press 500 pounds, but can do it 50 times in a row. Does the stronger athlete in this case have an advantage? No! The athlete with more muscular endurance has the advantage.

Once again we are talking about training the body to do the correct thing. Training is very work-specific; although there is some training carryover from one sport to another. When muscle endurance is important for sport, it must be achieved in sport-specific training, and training must be done at or near competition speeds.

The coach must know what muscles are involved in the sport and how to train them specifically so the athlete can perform maximally and at the same time avoid injury.

Power Endurance

Power endurance is the ability to repeatedly perform a skill with adequate speed, and is usually measured by the number of repetitions an athlete can perform within a set time limit. Long-term power endurance training will improve the muscles' ability to use oxygen, thereby increasing endurance.

Reaction Time

Reaction time is the time elapsed between a stimulus and the start of movement. An example here would be the batter in baseball who has to decide whether or not to swing at the ball. The time spent processing and signaling is called reaction time. It is doubtful that signaling time can be improved, but with practice and experience, the processing time can be improved.

Quickness

Quickness can be thought of as the way an athlete reacts within a small area (one or two steps). An athlete's initial speed depends on muscular power and the athlete with a high level of muscular power can accelerate quickly in order to make necessary adjustments within a small area (one or two steps).

Speed

Speed is the final result of reaction time and quickness combined. Sports such as hockey, volleyball, and linemen in football require good reaction time and quickness, while other sports such as soccer, lacrosse, and receivers in football require speed as well.

One athlete may not be as fast as another athlete. But if the slower athlete can react faster and get from one spot to another quicker he or she has an advantage. Does every athlete on a team have the same amount of strength? Of course not! You need to put the athlete you are working with in position to use the strength, power, muscular endurance and speed they have to their individual advantage.

Flexibility

Flexibility is the range of motion through which a joint is able to move. This will depend not only on gender (male or female), but on the design of the joint and the associated muscles, tendons and ligaments. It is important to remember that more is not necessarily better. This means that as athletes extend their flexibility beyond what is needed for their sport, the joint can become less stable and may become more prone to injury.

Agility

Agility is the ability to rapidly change direction and speed, with accuracy, and without loss of balance. This will depend on strength, power, power endurance, speed, reaction time, quickness, balance and flexibility.

It is very important to practice sport-specific movements. Playing in games requiring rapid changes of direction such as racquetball, handball and tennis during the off-season can help improve agility.

Muscular strength, cardiovascular endurance, muscle endurance and flexibility all play a part in health, fitness and sports performance. Sports-specific performance is a lot different from training for health and fitness, and better sports performance is not always related to good health. An overall conditioning program, addressing each fitness component is important.

Training to Jump Higher

Athletes are always telling me they want to jump higher. There is a simple way to improve vertical jump and vertical jump quickness. Cut a tambourine (12-15" circle) out of a piece of plywood. Drill a hole in the center and string a rope up through it (knot at the end of the rope so the rope will not pull through). Run the rope up over a beam (using a pulley) so you can adjust the height.

Have the athlete stand under the tambourine and have them jump off both feet as high as they can so they can outreach the tambourine by about an inch. Now have the athlete jump 10 consecutive times, rebounding without pause, attempting to touch the tambourine 10 consecutive times. If the athlete misses before the 10th time have them stop and walk around for a minute or two, to replace the ATP, and then try again. As soon as the athlete can touch the tambourine 10 consecutive times, raise it up another inch and start again.

Do this drill twice a week and watch what happens! Their vertical jump will increase 1-6 inches in a very short amount of time. You may end up with an athlete who can't jump as high as one of his or her teammates but can actually jump quicker; which may be more important to their particular sport. You are training a specific system to do a specific thing.

Designing an Exercise Program

One of the great ways to help athletes today is sport specificity training; duplicating the actual motions of a sport against resistance.

Have you ever heard this statement: "Do 3 sets of 10, or 3 sets of 12 or 15?" When I visit health clubs I will often ask people "what are you doing?" And they say 3 sets of 10; I say, "Why? Why not do one set of 30 and go home?" They usually have no idea. Are you training strength, power, quickness, endurance or some combination? Are you training the ATP/PC, Lactic Acid, Glycogen, or Fat system, or some combination? Are you training fast or slow twitch muscles? If you don't know and understand what you are doing how can you expect to have positive results? You can't!

To develop strength the athlete needs to work as many muscle fibers at one time as possible. This is done by lifting heavy weights and low repetitions. To develop muscular endurance you lift lighter weight with more repetitions. What is important to consider is that strength in and of itself does not guarantee success. The strongest football player on a team may not be the best player because he may lack the speed, agility, balance and coordination necessary and can be outmaneuvered and out leveraged despite his strength.

The two different types of competitive lifting require different elements: In Power lifting (bench press, squat, dead lift) speed is not a key element. But in Olympic lifting (clean and jerk, the snatch) explosive speed is critical. Good examples of power are the first step in basketball, changing directions in football or coming out of starting blocks in track.

QUICKNESS: Involves several different factors:

Strength - the more force you can generate the greater your speed.

Resistance - weights, your own body, or an object (shot put, javelin).

Nerve Stimulation - speed of movement is affected by the speed of nerve impulses.

Fast/Slow Twitch Muscle Fibers – remember you cannot change the ratio of fast to slow twitch fibers but you can maximize the development of fast twitch fibers with proper weight training. Research tells us that you are born with a ratio of fast to slow twitch fibers. You can, however, increase the size and capacity of both fast and slow twitch fibers by different types of training.

Biomechanics - putting your body in the correct position can increase speed.

Anticipation - thinking about the movement before you do it can help the nervous system respond.

Types of Exercise (reviewed):

Isometric

Pushing or pulling against an immovable object. In this form of exercise muscle tension is increased but there is little or no change in muscle length. The majority of research suggests that contractions of 3 to 10 seconds, with a low number of repetitions done on a daily basis works best.

Isotonic

During this type of training there is a change in the length of the muscle. Lifting free weights is the classic form of isotonic exercise. Increases in strength for both sexes due to this type of training are well documented.

Eccentric:

Often called negative resistance, it means that the muscle actually lengthens during the contraction. Lifting of a weight causes the muscle to shorten as it contracts and is called a concentric contraction. Muscle tension is higher during eccentric contractions than it is during either isometric or isotonic contractions which can lead to the development of greater post-exercise soreness.

Variable:

This type of equipment operates through a lever arm, cam, or pulley arrangement that allows the altering of resistance throughout the range of motion.

<u>**Isokinetic**</u>:

A method by which the resistance is increased during the lift proportional to whatever force you apply to it. An advantage is that it allows for speeds of contraction closer to speeds encountered during athletic performance while producing minimal muscle and joint soreness.

<u>**Isorobic**</u>:

This method combines isometrics with isotonic and variable resistance to give a very efficient method of exercise. In addition it is very efficient for sports-specificity training. I have been using this method personally since 1963 and highly recommend it. Go to my personal web site (www.JackMedina.com) and take a good look at this program (click on link: "Jack Recommends") watch my demonstration of the exercises and see why I recommend it so highly for virtually everyone at all ages. Call my office at 1-866-204-8786 if you have any questions.

Each of the above types of exercise has its advantages and disadvantages but the majority of research indicates there is no significant difference in gains made from any of the various methods. The key is the coach having knowledge in each of these areas and how to apply them based upon the equipment available to his athletes and time available for training.

If you were going to design a strength program for the chest as an example, using Isotonic exercise, I would have the athlete lay on a bench and find out how much weight can put on the bar so he can do 10 repetitions but not number 11. This is his 10 repetition maximum. Once this has been established with each exercise the training can begin.

I usually have the athlete start at 50% of this 10 RM maximum and do 15 repetitions as a warm-up. After a 30-90 second rest period, during which the athlete drinks some water, the athlete now starts the first set, just barely finishing the 10th repetition. Another 30-90 second rest period (with water) and the second set is done; however it is not possible to do 10 repetitions, maybe 7 or 8 at the most. Another 30-90 second rest (with water) and the third set is completed with maybe 5-6 repetitions. A 30-90 second rest period (with water) followed by 15 repetitions at 50% of the 10 RM max working through a full range of motion for flexibility and warm-down.

As soon as the athlete can do three sets of 10 repetitions it is time to increase the intensity of the exercise by adding more weight, adding repetitions, changing angles of the exercise (wide grip to narrow grip, barbell to dumbbell, standing to sitting, etc.) or working against the clock depending upon what you are working on: strength, power, quickness or endurance. These changes in your exercise program should occur somewhere between 8 and 12 weeks on a regular basis.

REMEMBER THE FOLLOWING:

- Every time the angle of an exercise is changed, the exercise changes.

- It used to be that training programs consisted of performing large group exercises prior to exercising the smaller muscle groups. More recently, different types of methods have been used which reverse the order. As an example, doing leg extensions prior to squats or lat pulls prior to bench presses. Using a variety of different methods helps avoid boredom in your routine.

- Typically, 3 to 6 sets are used to achieve significant gains in strength. However, use of 1 or 2 sets of an exercise may be more appropriate for beginners in the initial stages of a base program (first 6-12 workouts).

- Because the ATP-PC energy source is the most powerful, it is required during maximal or near-maximal sets. When training this energy source, at least 2-3 minutes of rest between sets is necessary. This rest period dictates the amount of stress put on the lactic acid energy source since if the rest period is less than one minute, plasma lactic acid concentrations are extremely high.

- If lactic acid is identified as a primary energy source, the rest periods may be shortened to allow the buildup of plasma lactic acid. This encourages an increased tolerance of more acidic conditions which may benefit the anaerobic (without oxygen) athlete such as wrestlers, gymnasts, sprinters (100 to 800 meters), basketball, football and baseball players.

One of the really good references for details in weight training is the book "Getting Stronger" by Bill Pearl and Gary T. Moran, PhD.

Also remember that one form of exercise does not always carry over to another one. Example, you are in really good shape for playing basketball, and then you go play a different sport or do a different activity and are sore the next day. Why are you sore? It's because the muscles used for one activity are different than those used in a different one; therefore there is some connective tissue tearing and you will be sore until the healing takes place.

Weights vs. Machines:

Both have their advantages and disadvantages. Free weights often allow for more sport-specific training and allow for muscle groups involved in balance and body stabilization. Machines are generally safer and easier to use for beginners. Machines also help to stabilize the body, reduce balance problems and isolate movement to main muscle groups.

If I had to make a choice I would use free weights because free weights develop balance, coordination and a degree of strength not possible in training on machines. Using free weights also helps train concentration, which is extremely valuable in any sport. When the athlete has to balance as well as lift the weight, they must focus their undivided attention on the exercise.

Free Weights - are the most commonly used type of weightlifting equipment in the world. The two major pieces are barbells and dumbbells along with auxiliary equipment like flat benches, incline benches, decline benches, and pullover benches. This stationary equipment allows you to change your body position so you can work all the muscles from different angles with barbells or dumbbells.

Traditional Machines - like the lat machine, quad pulley, leg extension, seated rowing machine, etc. have been around for decades.

Universal and Similar Type Machines - these are good because up to 14 people can work on a multi-station Universal machine at one time. They are excellent for the beginner to start weight training and are easy to use. These machines are safer to use than free weights because there is no risk of plates slipping off bars and no risk of being pinned by the weights. Disadvantages include a narrow range of individual movements, and you cannot work the body from numerous angles as you can with free weights.

Nautilus Machines - and other Isokinetic machines are said to exercise the muscles evenly throughout the complete range of motion, which free weights do not do. Because of this feature you can get an intense workout quickly and it is safer than free weights (they have stretching built into the movement) and you can't drop something on yourself. Disadvantages: the machine provides the balance and you don't develop the same ligament or tendon strength in the joints as you do with free weights, and since Nautilus isolates muscles, you don't work as many muscles at one time. Nautilus machines do not teach coordination and only 2 or 3 movements can be done for each body part which can eventually lead to boredom.

Training Belts - These belts have a wide portion on the back that supposedly helps support the lower back (lumbar area). Yes, these belts do support the low back, but not because of the wide back area, but rather because it gives the abdominal muscles an object to push against.

A training belt, though it isn't necessary for safe performance, can be used for exercises that place a lot of stress on the lower back, such as squats and dead lifts. It should not be used to compensate for technique problems caused by weak abdominal or low back musculature. If the exercise being done is going to place a significant amount of stress on the low back, exercises to strengthen the low back should be included in the training program.

Wearing a training belt that is cinched tightly during an activity increases blood pressure which can put undue stress on the cardiovascular system; so don't wear one during exercises that are not going to significantly stress the low back, such as riding a stationary bicycle. Training belts should not be worn when performing exercises that do not require back support or use light to moderate resistance.

Plyometrics - This method of exercise, (stretch-shortening) is thought of as performing body weight jumping-type movements such as jumping off an object, and immediately up onto another object (depth jump) and throwing medicine balls. For example, during walking, every time the foot hits the ground, the quadriceps (thigh muscles) goes through this stretch-shortening cycle; the muscle is stretched slightly and then shortens. The slight stretching stores elastic energy which explains why a more forceful concentric action results. Many medicine ball exercises for the upper body involve this stretch-shortening cycle. The depth jump is probably most often associated with this stretch-shortening cycle, but virtually all jump exercises and throwing exercises, where there is no pause in the movement, involve this "plyometric" principle of exercise.

Testing for Muscular Fitness

The first question to ask is WHY this particular test? To be of value, both to a coach and to the athlete, it must be useful. In order to be useful it must meet several criteria:

1. It MUST be sport-specific and valid - it must measure what it is designed to measure.

2. Reliable - must be repeatable.

3. Objective - is not affected by a coach's bias.

4. Gender and age appropriate.

5. Easy for athletes to learn.

6. Easy to administer.

7. Provide results that can be used to monitor progress.

Before any testing is done, athletes should be well rested, and as soon as possible after tests are administered, athletes should be given feedback regarding strengths, areas of weakness, and areas for improvement.

TRAINING SYSTEMS

Strength Training/Resistance Training, as opposed to weight training which generally refers to the use of free weights (barbells & dumbbells), can include a wide range of activities and equipment. Strength training can use a person's own body-weight to improve strength such as push-ups, sit-ups, dips, chin-ups, etc. Many programs can also use other forms of equipment such as sandbags, tires, elastic bands, and chains as the resistance. In my opinion the primary purpose of strength training is to prevent injury and improve performance potential. Proper strength training will help keep you in shape on a year-round basis.

If you look at the various fitness magazines and muscle magazines you will see a wide variety of training methods. Is one absolutely better than another one? Probably not! The best exercise program ever developed is the one you will use. There are many different opinions as to which system is best and more research is being done all the time. I have tried to include realistic information in this section that you can use as an athlete or as someone who just wants to get into shape physically. There is something for everyone. Not only the athlete who wants to improve his or her performance but for those people who use the typical excuses of **time, boredom, soreness, convenience, and lack of motivation** for not working out. For these people, the section on "Isorobics" should really benefit you.

Individualizing Exercise Prescriptions

People will often ask their instructor or coach, "Is there a good weight-training program for me?" This question is asked because it is not uncommon for people to believe that there is a magic program which will result in unbelievable strength gains. To a certain extent this may be true because consistent training with proper variation and adherence to a well-designed program, with proper basic principles of training being followed, will allow for optimal gains in strength according to each individual's genetic potential. This is an important factor for consideration and is often overlooked.

As a person starts a training program, the initial gains are usually great because of the large potential to be realized. As training moves forward, gains slow down as the individual approaches his or her potential.

Each exercise program must be designed according to individual specifications such as their fitness level. One of the most common mistakes made in designing a workout program is placing too much stress on the individual before he or she can tolerate it. An individual begins a training session with a certain amount of strength. As the session progresses there is a loss of strength due to fatigue; and at the end of the session strength is at its lowest point. After recovering from the first workout session the individual should begin the next workout at a slightly higher strength level. This is called a staircase effect and should be repeated for each training session. This is the biggest challenge for trainers in the field of resistance training.

Major design components reviewed:

- **Needs Analysis** - answering some initial questions:

  a. What muscle groups need to be trained?
  b. What are the basic energy sources which need to be trained (anaerobic, aerobic)?
  c. What type of muscle action (isometric, variable, isotonic, etc.) should be used?
  d. What are primary sites of injury for the particular sport (if it is a sports related program design)?

- **Acute Program Variables** - every time the angle of an exercise changes, the exercise changes. Various exercises can also be classified as structural or body part. Structural are those lifts requiring the coordinated action of many muscle groups. Power cleans, power snatches, dead lifts, and squats are good examples. Exercises which try to isolate a particular muscle group are considered body-part exercises. Bicep curls, sit ups, and leg curls are good examples here. It is important to include structural exercises when whole body strength movements are required for a particular sport. This is the case for activities such as football, basketball, wrestling, and track and field.

  For individuals interested in basic fitness, these exercises are advantageous only when there is a limited amount of time and it is necessary to train more than one muscle group at a time.

- **Order of Exercise** - for many years the order of exercise in resistive training consisted of performing large muscle group exercises prior to performing the smaller muscle groups. More recently, different types of methodology have been used which reverse the order, exercising smaller muscle groups prior to large muscle groups. An example of this would be doing leg extensions followed by squats, or doing lat pull-downs followed by bench presses. You should be aware of the fact that the advantage of one type of training, large muscle groups followed by small muscle groups or visa versa has yet to be demonstrated.

- **Number of Sets** - the number of sets used in a workout is directly related to training results. Typically, three to six sets are used to achieve significant gains in strength. It has been suggested that using multiple sets works best for developing strength and local muscular endurance. However, the use of one or two sets of an exercise may be more appropriate for beginners in the initial stages of a basic program.

- **Rest Periods** - because the ATP-PC energy source is the most powerful it is required during maximal or near-maximal sets such as one to three or four repetition maximums. The amount of rest between sets and exercises also dictates the amount of stress placed on the lactic acid energy source. When rest periods are less than one minute long, plasma lactic acid concentrations are extremely high. This is also true in circuit training where relatively light loads of 40% to 60% of one-repetition maximums are used. Lactic acid's involvement in fatigue has been the subject of much controversy. The length of the rest period will determine to a great extent the amount of lactic acid which is produced and removed from the body.

  If the needs analysis identifies lactic acid as the primary energy source, the rest periods can be gradually shortened to allow the buildup of plasma lactic acid, encouraging an increased tolerance to more acidic conditions. This type of training may be best for such anaerobic athletes as wrestlers, sprinters, basketball players, and football players.

Training Systems

Olympic lifters, power lifters or body builders originally developed most resistance/strength training systems being used today. They are popular today because they produce increases in strength and muscular growth (hypertrophy), or because a particular system has been promoted by a particular company or individual; not because they have been scientifically proven to be superior. There is still a great deal of controversy as to whether or not one system is that much superior to any other system. More research is needed on all training methods or systems being used today.

Two common mistakes to avoid when designing a training program:

1. Don't assume that because a champion body builder, Olympic lifter or power lifter uses a given system that it is the best one, especially for the beginner. Many times these programs are too intense for newcomers. All individuals will make gains in strength when using resistive exercise but the "Champions" you see in the various magazines, etc. also have the genetic potential for superior strength and size.

2. Not having a training/progress record. This type of record can be extremely helpful in answering questions concerning a person's response to a training program. I can't tell you how many times I have asked to look at a training record and found that this person has been doing the same program for month upon month, has quit making progress and can't understand why. Programs should be evaluated on a regular 6-12 week basis in order to track progress and make changes when and where necessary, not only to continue challenging various muscle groups but also the individual who is training.

Free Weight Training Systems

If you are going to use free weights or machines for your training, here are a variety of different programs you might want to consider. I suggest you change your workout program every 6-12 weeks. This helps eliminate boredom and challenges new muscles tissue on a regular basis.

- **Single Sets** - doing one set of each exercise (8-15 repetitions). Significant gains in strength have been demonstrated using this method.

- **Multiple Sets** - this usually consists of a couple of warm-up sets of increasing resistance (adding some weight after each set) followed by several sets at the same resistance. Most research available today suggests that 5-8 repetitions performed for 3 sets appears to be best in terms of potential strength gains.

- **Light To Heavy** - this means progressing from a light to heavy resistance using a set of 5-8 repetitions for each exercise with a light weight, then adding 5 pounds and doing another set. Continue this until only one repetition can be performed.

- **Heavy to Light** - just the reverse of light to heavy. After a warm-up, the heaviest set is performed first and for each succeeding set the resistance is lowered.

- **Super Setting** - this is very popular with body builders. If your goal is primarily to increase muscle size, you might want to try super setting. There are two types, both using 8-10 repetitions with little or no rest in between repetitions or sets:

    1. Do several sets of two exercises for the same body part using two antagonistic muscles. Example: arm curls immediately followed by triceps extensions or, leg extensions immediately followed by leg curls.

    2. One set of several exercises all for the same body part. Example: Lat pull, seated rowing and bent over rowing (all for the back); or, squats, leg presses and leg curls.

- **Tri-Sets** - means using groups of 3 exercises for the same body part. Exercises include different muscle groups with little or no rest in between exercises or sets. Normally 3 sets of each exercise are performed. Example: arm curls, triceps extension, and military press (all emphasizing the arms). The short rest periods and the use of 3 exercises in series for one body part make this a good system to increase muscular endurance.

- **Circuit Training** - this is a series of exercises performed one after the other with 15 - 30 second rest periods between each exercise. Ten to 15 repetitions of each exercise are performed per circuit at 40-60% of a one repetition maximum. This type of training is very time efficient when large numbers of individuals are involved such as a class or members of a team. In fact, you can work against the clock, to raise the intensity, instead of doing a set number of repetitions. Example: see how many repetitions of each exercise you can do, with good form, in 30 seconds.

- **Split Routine** - this is time consuming and as a result all body parts cannot be exercised in a single training session. Different body parts are trained on alternate days. Example: Training the arms, legs and abdomen on Monday, Wednesday, Friday and chest, shoulders and back Tuesday, Thursday and Saturday. Eight to 10 repetitions are performed with a one-minute rest period between from 3 to 6 sets.

- **Cheat System** – this is a popular method of training among body builders. It means you are breaking strict form when doing an exercise. Example: When doing standing barbell curls, rather than maintaining a straight (vertical) upper body you use a slight body swing to start the barbell moving. Another example would be arching your back when attempting a bench press.

- **Exhaustion Program** – this is a one set 10 repetition to exhaustion system and can be incorporated into any of the other training methods. Those who recommend this method believe more motor units will be recruited, thus receiving a training stimulus, than when sets are not done to exhaustion.

- **The Burn** – an extension of the exhaustion system. It can also be used with any of the training systems. After a set of an exercise is performed to exhaustion, 5-6 half or partial repetitions are done which cause an aching or burning sensation.

- **Multi-Poundage** - This requires spotters to assist you, never ever try this by yourself. One person does 4-5 repetitions at a 4-5 maximum resistance. The spotters then remove 20-40 pounds of weight and another set of 4-5 repetitions are performed. This is continued for several sets.

- **Super Pump System** – this is for advanced lifters desiring greater muscle hypertrophy (size gains) of the arms, chest and shoulders. Those recommending this method of training believe that advanced body builders need to perform 15-18 sets for each body part per training session. Anywhere from 1-3 exercises per muscle group are performed per training session with a 15 second rest period between sets of 5-6 repetitions. Correct form is very important and each muscle group is trained 2-3 times per week. This method seems to be most beneficial for the development of the chest, arms and shoulders; it is too fatiguing to use in training the back and legs.

- **Functional Isometrics** - this involves performing a static (Dynamic) contraction at the "sticking point" of an exercise. Example: often-times during bench presses you can press the bar only part way up (sticking point). The objective here is to use Isometrics to cause a gain in strength at the weakest point in the range of motion; usually a 3-10 second contraction.

As you can see from the above training methods, there is wide variety in weight training today. If you are going to use weight training (free weights or machines) you can select from many different methods. Select the one that fits your particular needs and time schedule.

GETTING STRONGER!

Earlier we mentioned the "overload" principal, which is the key to getting stronger. In resistance training, a muscle, or groups of muscles can be overloaded in a number of ways:

1. Adding more resistance.

2. Increasing the number of repetitions.

3. Changing the speed of movement.

4. Increasing the frequency of workouts.

5. Changing the angle (wide grip to narrow grip, barbell to dumbbell, standing to sitting, or through some combination of the above.

When using these techniques, remember that conditioning programs should involve muscle groups directly related to their use in a sport or activity.

Methods of Resistance Training:

These are generally divided into three categories:

1. *Isometrics* or static contractions - these are contractions against an immovable object. However, there are few benefits to be gained using this method because most sports require dynamic, not static strength. Static contractions still have value, but only in activities or sports that use this type of contraction, such as shooting, archery, or rock climbing.

2. *Isotonics*, or same-weight resistance training - the same weight is lifted through a range of motion. This is often called "dynamic constant external resistance." This type of training involves both concentric and eccentric muscle contractions. Concentric contractions occur when the muscle shortens during the lift, and eccentric contraction occurs when the muscle lengthens as the load is lowered. Research supports using a combination of these methods, however, eccentric contractions are known to produce excessive muscle soreness when the overload is increased too rapidly—it must be done gradually.

3. *Isokinetics*, or same-speed, variable-resistance training makes sense. This method, done at the speeds required for a given sport, provide for optimal sport-specific overload. Research has shown that athletes who train at high speeds can generate better power at high-movement speeds than athletes who train at low speeds.

Isokinetic training:

1. Is ideally suited for performance of exercise at velocities similar to those required in specific sports.

2. Provides a training effect through a complete range of motion.

3. Generally involves concentric contractions and does not produce a lot of muscle soreness.

Training Terms & Tips:

Muscle Balance - each sport has its primary movers called "agonists"; these are the major muscle sources required for movement. It is easy to design training programs for these, but don't forget about the opposing muscle "agonists"; example, quadriceps vs. hamstring.

Repetition Maximum - the number of times a load can be lifted before exhaustion. If an athlete can lift a weight 10 times before exhaustion, this is his or her 10-repetition maximum (10 RM load).

Sets, Repetitions, Circuits:

1. A *repetition* is one complete cycle of an exercise, such as one curl or bench press or sit-up.

2. A *set* is the number of repetitions completed without a rest period.

3. *Circuit training* means putting sets of exercises together without repeating the same exercise twice in a row. Example: one set of 10 dips, then push-ups, bench presses, curls, etc. This kind of training is popular for power endurance development.

4. *Set/rep Training* - uses multiple repeated sets of one exercise before the next exercise is done; such as 3 sets of 10 bench presses followed by 3 sets of squats.

Intensity - generally refers to the number of repetitions to failure or percent of maximum (1 repetition maximum).

Rest Period - the amount of recovery time between sets or exercises.

Core Stability - the role of core muscles (trunk, hips, and shoulders) in stabilizing the primary movers of the limbs. Strength coaches need to recognize the importance of having a strong base from which to develop sport power. By first stabilizing the abdominal, back, and shoulder muscles, the athlete will increase their training gains, improve performance, and reduce low back and other injuries. Core exercises usually involve 15 or 30 repetitions.

Exercise Order - may have a large impact on gains in strength, power and power endurance. Multiple joint exercises, such as the squat, are effective for increasing general muscular strength, and focus should be on these exercises for optimal muscular strength improvement. Start with multiple-joint exercises early in training and then progress towards sport-specific exercises as the competitive season approaches.

1. Begin with light warm-up sets for all muscle groups.

2. Train large muscle groups first before small groups and multiple joint exercises before single-joint exercises, and high-intensity exercises before low-intensity exercises.

Velocity - performing resistance training at moderate speeds produces reasonable strength gains while slow movements, due to high resistance, are great for developing strength. Moderate and fast velocities have been shown to develop better power. Untrained athletes should start with slow velocities and moderate resistance and then move to moderate and higher velocities as technique and strength improves.

Keys to Getting Stronger

The length of time necessary to develop strength may require as much as 6-12 weeks or longer. During the first 6-8 weeks there probably will be little if any muscle hypertrophy (growth). After 6-8 weeks, increases in strength will primarily be the result of muscle growth, along with metabolic improvements. Endurance athletes, who want increases in strength, but not muscle mass, should limit their strength training to about 8-10 weeks to avoid muscle growth.

For the untrained person, muscular improvements can be seen with as little as 50% of a one repetition maximum or a weight they can lift or move 15 to 20 times. However, the basic recommendation is to use a resistance of 60-70% of a one repetition maximum for 8-12 repetitions. For advanced athletes, they can use 80 - 100% of 1 RM; however, using a variety of resistance is more effective than when the same resistance is used for all sets.

Developing Power

It is important to understand that power is the result of applying force quickly. You have to develop strength before you can develop power. For ultimate performance, almost all sports require increases in power. Research has shown that power training, using light to moderate workloads at high velocities, is more effective in increasing sports-specific power; the problem is the ballistic nature of machines and free weights during the concentric (shortening) phase of the exercise. New machines, which allow for explosive movement, are being developed but some traditional exercises, like loaded jump squats, are possible for improving vertical jump.

Developing Power Endurance

It is difficult to categorize every sport into specific strength, power, or endurance events; most include all aspects of muscular and energy fitness to some degree. For power endurance it is critical to duplicate, as much as possible, the speed and motion used in the sport. Both strength and power training will improve power endurance to some extent. However, more repetitions and specificity of training will produce the best results. A basketball player should consider multiple vertical jumps wearing weight vests; sprinters pull weight using a running harness; distance runners may do repeat distances uphill; and swimmers may do tethered swimming.

How Many Sets?

Research shows that both single and multiple sets are similar in efficiency for athletes starting a resistance exercise program. As strength improves, the training volume needs to increase to two to four sets. The rest between sets is important (60-90 seconds). As intensity increases, rest periods should increase. No matter what sport it is, strength training will lay the foundation for power, which is an absolute must in all sports.

Maintaining Muscular Strength

In general, the higher your fitness level, the more training necessary to maintain that level. But to compete effectively you need rest and a reduction in training volume; as a result, this reduction or "tapering" will allow adequate rest. About two resistance training sessions per week are usually adequate to maintain preseason strength gains.

Muscle Balance

This refers to opposing muscles or muscle groups being balanced between primary movers and antagonist muscles (those causing the opposite movement).

Speed

Speed means acceleration from a starting position and implies power; maintaining speed requires muscle endurance. Thus, the athlete needs power to accelerate to speeds necessary for performance success; depending on the sport or event, power endurance may be required to maintain this speed.

Though genetics play a role in determining speed potential, all athletes can improve their acceleration, maximal and sub-maximal speeds. The ratio of fast to slow twitch fibers might not change during training, but the physiology of the cells can improve, resulting increased endurance and power.

Training for Speed

An athlete who spends the most time practicing at the speeds necessary for success is most likely to be able to perform at that speed during competition.

Keys for improving speed:

1. Be patient - developing speed takes time.

2. The athlete needs to rest between intervals during training so he or she can maintain speed. They should do as many intervals as possible as long as the speed is maintained.

3. Athletes need to be rested prior to speed training days. Thus speed work should follow easy days of training.

SPORT-SPECIFIC TRAINING

It is important for coaches and athletes to understand basic components of energy systems (covered earlier in this chapter) as well as the demands of the specific activity or sport. Athletes need to be trained specifically for their event or position. A great deal of this training should depend upon the energy system or systems are being used.

Anaerobic Training:

In sports requiring maximal or near-maximal force production (heavy lifts, sprints, etc.), most of the energy is provided by stored ATP and PC. Will creatine supplementation help? Recent studies have demonstrated the short-term effects of creatine supplementation—the ability to do more sets and repetitions during weight training. Unfortunately, the long-term effects have not received adequate study. Will the ability to do more sets and repetitions carry over to performance? This has not been proven, and until it is, why take the risks? (See the Supplement section).

Aerobic Training:

The effects of aerobic training are dramatic, clear and specific; it increases blood volume to the muscle, the number of capillaries serving each muscle fiber, and positively effects the cardiovascular and respiratory systems. Aerobic training can also increase the amount of fat (triglyceride) stored in muscle and the ability to burn fat. When fat is used as a primary source of energy, limited amounts of muscle and liver glycogen are conserved. The ability of the trained muscle to use fat may be the most important health benefit of aerobic fitness. If you are aerobically fit, you use fat during both rest and recovery, allowing the muscle to store more glycogen. By burning fat you reduce the likelihood that it will be deposited in adipose tissue (in places you don't want it) or in the coronary arteries, leading to the number one killer, heart disease. All of this has enormous implications for both endurance and health.

Training Program Guidelines:

Each sport has specific muscular and energy requirements. Here are some examples:

Athletes in skill sports, such as golf, table tennis, shooting, and bowling, improve dramatically with proper physical training and this improves distance and consistency while reducing the risk of over-use injuries.

In power sports, such as a football lineman, it requires a high level of muscular strength and power, particularly in the muscle groups involved in blocking and tackling. These movements require a strong core, as well as leg, neck, arm, and shoulders.

The most advanced in football training has been the addition of power training: force at high speed. This contributes to the ability to fire off the ball and drive an opponent. Football is a series of anaerobic efforts, each lasting 4-10 seconds followed by a recovery period lasting about 25 seconds. The increase in size of linemen has increased the need for aerobic and anaerobic energy training. Aerobic power will enhance the ability to recover between plays, thus improving performance, especially late in a game.

An example of a power endurance sport is wrestling and judo, which is the application of force and speed together. Because the competition lasts only a few minutes, wrestlers and judokas' need short to medium term power endurance and must be prepared to sustain a total effort for several minutes. Both the upper and lower body, as well as core muscles for controlling, lifting and throwing an opponent must be trained. Wrestling and judo bouts put a major demand on the anaerobic energy system, but both need good aerobic ability to assist in recovery, not only between periods, but during day long tournaments.

Start and go sports such as soccer, basketball, field hockey, and lacrosse consist of bursts of energy with periods of less demanding effort. Muscular fitness is needed to maximize power and speed and to withstand contact with opposing players. A strong aerobic foundation is needed in order to maintain continuous motion and to recover quickly between bursts of activity. Skills must be practiced at game speed if they are to be successful in competition.

Aerobic sports, such as cross country running, requires exceptional aerobic power. Any event lasting more than 15 minutes gets 80% of the energy from aerobic pathways, so training should emphasize race-pace training. Some anaerobic training should be done to build leg speed and the ability to kick at the end of a race. A considerable amount of time in the easy training zone is necessary to develop endurance and to allow recovery from more intense training. The goal with resistance training is not to build muscle, but rather strength to improve power endurance. Studies show that runners with good technique can out-perform opponents even when the opponent has an edge on aerobic power. Because of this, work should be done to enhance arm swing and natural stride.

THE PERFECT PROGRAM

Is there a perfect exercise program? Probably not! I think this will vary from individual to individual, so finding a perfect program for everyone would be futile. But, there are common elements in a well-designed program that will fit regardless of age, ability, and level of training because the basics of resistance/strength training have not changed over the years. After I go over these basics I'll attempt to show you what I think personally is as close to the "perfect" program as you can get.

First Step: Know Your Blood Pressure

You don't need a physician in order to get this test done. You can go to your local pharmacy, Wal-Mart, Target, or K-Mart, and purchase an easy to use unit. Many stores now have a blood pressure testing station where you simply slide your arm into a cuff, press the "start" button and everything is done for you.

Once you have the cuff in place, pump the pressure up (unless it is automatic) to 180 mm of pressure. As the pressure is released you will either see the light flash or hear a beep, or both. This represents your "systolic" blood pressure—pressure in the artery as blood leaves the heart. When the light stops flashing, or the beeping stops, this is the "diastolic" pressure, and represents the pressure as blood returns to your heart. Normal blood pressure is 120/80 or lower.

If the systolic (higher) number is 140 or more, or the diastolic (lower) number is 90 or higher, I suggest you check with your physician. This is the only way you have of looking inside our own body and blood pressure should be checked once each month.

After taking the tests mentioned, plus taking your body measurements to see where you are, you should be motivated to make some changes. I recommend measuring the amount of inches around your stomach at the navel (or the largest point in the abdominal or hip area that you can consistently find), around the mid-thigh (mid-point between the bend at the top outer part of the leg and your knee), and around the mid-arm (mid-point between your elbow and the bone at the top outer part of your shoulder). These should provide good "check-points" of your progress.

Types of Exercise

If you are going to exercise, there are only two methods: moving or not moving! If you are not moving it is "static" meaning **Isometric**. This method develops strength but has virtually no effect on flexibility or the heart.

If you're moving, you are using one of four types of exercise. **Isotonics** (movement) which relates primarily to resistance exercise. As a weight begins to move it gets lighter, which isn't ideal.

The second type of movement exercise is **Isokinetics**, which means the speed and resistance is controlled throughout the motion. Most of the equipment that applies this method is very expensive.

The third type of movement exercise is **Aerobic**—any exercise which works the cardiovascular system.

The fourth type of movement exercise is **Isorobic**, a combination of the best concepts available today (discussed at the end of this section). I highly recommend this program because it eliminates all the excuses for not exercising.

What is the best time to exercise? *When you are in your shorts or less, or when it fits into your time schedule.*

Basic one - Repetitions! Though there is some disagreement here, the general consensus says that the most beneficial repetition includes a concentric phase (the muscle shortens) in which the weight is raised and an eccentric phase (the muscle lengthens) in which the weight is lowered. Can strength improvements occur when only raising and not lowering a weight? Yes! This has been proved dramatically in using the Isorobic concept as the basis for training. However, when using typical weight training machines or "free weights", raising and lowering of the resistance is generally accepted.

Basic Two - Resistance! This can be most anything from the most complicated machine to a tire, bale of hay, elastic band, human partner or your own body (push-ups, chin-ups, sit-ups, etc). The key is to use a resistance that develops tension within the muscle creating an overload factor. A muscle cannot discriminate between one source of tension and another source; any object that applies resistance that is appropriate can stimulate a training response.

Basic Three - Train the Whole Body - you really don't want to leave a specific muscle or area of the body untrained. All of the major muscle groups of the body should be trained (quadriceps, hamstrings, calves, hips, abdominals, back, shoulders, chest, arms).

Basic Four - Balance! You want to train both sides of a joint. Since a muscle can only contract, it can't lengthen with force; each joint generally has at least two or more muscle groups that make movement possible around that joint. These muscles, along with the connective tissue (ligaments and tendons) around the joint maintain its stability. However, **don't think that you can use an equal amount of resistance in both directions because there are biomechanical reasons why you may have more strength in one direction than in another** (i.e. quadriceps vs. hamstrings).

It is important to consider a balanced training approach not only between upper and lower body, but also right and left sides of the body.

If you will consider the above four basic elements when developing a resistive/strength training program you can eliminate a lot of "hype" about one system being better than another system. Let me emphasize once again, the best training program available today is ultimately the one you will do!

Key Elements to Check:

- Use a full range of motion for each exercise. The exception would be if you are using the "cheat" system.

- Eliminate jerky, fast movements when starting an exercise. It is possible to lift more weight by jerking the resistance because it ignores the basic principle of neurophysiology and specificity of muscle fiber recruitment.

- Try to reach muscular fatigue in the number of repetitions you are doing; the point at which another repetition is not possible.

- If you can, train under supervision or with a partner. This may not be possible in all circumstances.

Training Specificity - Ken Manni, Strength and Conditioning Coach at Michigan State University and a highly respected friend of mine indicates this is a much-misused term. He says, "Specificity can be put into perspective when you understand that the more complex the skill, the greater the importance of exactness when practicing it. In other words, the closer the influence of practice on the competition or sports situation, the better these movements will be recalled during the actual game or performance. Simply put, practice sessions should be designed to duplicate the game or condition as often as possible."

The Best Program - obviously the athletes, those participating in sports are required to do those exercises the coach or instructor demand of them.

If you personally are looking for an exercise program I think you have to consider four potential problems that could prevent you from achieving your goal: **time, boredom, convenience, soreness and motivation**. Do I have to spend 45 minutes or more 3 days per week in order to get the results I want? Do I have to keep adding repetitions to my exercises as I get stronger (starting with 5 push-ups now and a year from now having to do 105 to get the same result)? Do I have to join a gym or club in order to exercise (which may be inconvenient time and travel wise)? Will I be so sore after one or two days that I can't move because it hurts? Will I be motivated to continue this exercise program?

This book has not been written with only athletes in mind. I work with people who can't walk, jog or run; people with bad backs, people in wheelchairs, people who can't get down on the floor to exercise, people that can't get on or off exercise machines, people that can't travel to a workout facility, etc. It has been written for you!

As I travel worldwide speaking professionally I always indicate to audiences that the real key to success is YOU! I may want you to eat the right food, drink plenty of water and exercise regularly; but it doesn't matter what I want you to do, it only matters what you want to do. Maybe you should take this simple test:

Go into your bedroom all by yourself, shut and lock the door behind you, turn on every light in the room, remove all of your clothes, stand in from of a full length mirror and see if you like what you see. Allow 15 minutes for trauma to set in and you may finally be ready to go to work!

The four problems mentioned earlier, time, boredom, convenience, soreness and lack of motivation are the four excuses I hear regularly for not exercising. Over the past 4 decades that I have been involved in teaching and coaching, the exercise concept I recommend most is called ISOROBIC! Why? Because it takes the best of the exercise concepts available and combines them so the excuses people use for not exercising can be eliminated. It is a program that is portable (you can take it with you anywhere you go), is great for kids, adults and athletes alike, the concept has been researched and used in the NASA space program and, results are fast. What more can you ask for?

What concepts are combined?

- **Isometrics** - static contraction. Pulling or pushing against an immovable object. The maximum effect occurs at 10 seconds; there is no additional benefit after 10 seconds. This concept builds lactic acid within the blood quickly thus causing muscle fatigue. This eliminates a lot of repetitions, which in turn eliminates the boredom of doing the same exercise over and over.

- **Isotonics** - movement against resistance; which is great for developing strength through a full range of motion; which in turn enhances flexibility.

- **Isokinetics** - the ability to control speed and resistance throughout the exercise.

- **Aerobics** - the ability to increase the efficiency of the heart muscle.

I personally think that some form of resistance/strength training is important in any exercise program. I have personally participated in weight training and bodybuilding and have really enjoyed it. However, as a busy lifestyle began to interfere with my workout schedule, I found the Isorobic concept allowed me to stay in shape with a minimum amount of time spent; plus it made it convenient to train while I travel.

The Isorobic concept is very safe, including those people with bad backs, and the basic exercises can be done standing or sitting. I have used this concept with all of my athletes ages 7 through Olympic and professional for the past 38 years.

If you are interested in looking and feeling better, reducing body fat while increasing lean muscle mass (which burns calories like crazy) and flexibility, want to make your back stronger (without lifting), want to have a tight firm rear end and tight firm legs, here is a program for you.

You might consider looking at this Isorobic concept of exercise. If you have a computer or access to the internet, you can go to my website at www.JackMedina.com (click on the "Jack Recommends" link), watch my video demonstration of the exercises, and then make your own decision. You can call me at 1-866-204-8786 if you have questions about the Isorobic Exercise Program.

QUESTIONS ABOUT RESISTANCE/STRENGTH TRAINING

1. If I want to become fast, should I do fast repetitions?

So far the best recommendations come from a study done in 1990 by Voit and Klausen showing that even though heavy resistance training by itself does not improve the speed of a skilled movement, it can enhance movement speed if it is combined with sport-specific training. In other words, practice sport specific skills.

2. What about Intensity of Training?

This ultimately relates to each person's ability to work hard, which usually means performing maximal voluntary contractions; in other words recruiting as many fibers as possible. However, maximal voluntary contraction doesn't necessarily mean a one-repetition maximum. It could refer to the last repetition of an 8, 10, 12, or 15 repetition maximum.

3. Is there a relationship between hormone levels, strength training, and training results?

Scientific research does not support the widely held belief that large muscle mass and muscle size resulting from strength training is related to high levels of testosterone. The role of growth hormone is still unclear. It is too early to assume that growth hormone increases the size and strength of muscles regardless of what you might read or hear. More research is needed before this question can be answered with certainty.

4. Does strength training affect the cardiovascular system?

Definitely! It has been shown to increase time to exhaustion for cardiac-rehab patients on the treadmill and stationary bicycle. It has been shown that strength training has the potential to increase endurance performance, particularly that requiring fast-twitch fiber recruitment.

5. Does strength training have an effect on cholesterol?

It is important to understand first that cholesterol has many important functions in the body. It is part of the cell membrane and nerve fibers and it is required for the production of steroid hormones, bile acids, and vitamin D.

The body produces (synthesizes) about 1,000 milligrams of cholesterol every day in addition to what is taken in each day in the food you eat. Sixty-five to seventy percent of the cholesterol in the body is produced by the body itself; the liver and small intestine mucous being the primary organs that produce it.

Several factors can influence cholesterol levels other than exercise, which is why some studies show that strength training has a positive effect on cholesterol and other studies show no effect at all. One of these factors is diet which some of the studies do not account for. Another factor is that some studies on weight training and cholesterol fail to consider that a person being evaluated may already have a low cholesterol level to start with. Thus the study would fail to show any positive training effect.

If your cholesterol levels are in a low to normal range prior to starting a strength training program, don't expect major changes from the training program. However, if you have a high percentage of body fat and high cholesterol levels, you can lose body fat by reducing your caloric intake while at the same time you consume a diet of 60-65% carbohydrates, 20-25% fat, and 12-15% protein.

At the same time you have to train hard enough to challenge your muscles and encourage muscle growth. Strength training can help any person achieve and maintain a healthy cardiovascular system.

6. What effect does strength training have on metabolism?

First, what is metabolism? Metabolism involves chemical changes that utilize energy and result in tissue and compound building or breakdown of substrates and release of energy. Simply put, it is energy produced by the body!

Three ways strength training can affect metabolism:

- Muscles, in order to lift heavy loads, need energy. The amount of metabolic increase is dependent on the amount of muscle mass used in an exercise and the resistance used. The energy expenditure (metabolic rate) has been estimated to vary from 5-10 calories per minute depending upon whether you are using small or large muscle groups. Greater resistance equals a greater number of calories being used.

- The number of calories burned after exercise is relatively small; however, the good news is that after a workout more fat is used than carbohydrate to meet the energy needs of the body. The more carbohydrates used during the exercise, the more fat used afterward.

- High intensity strength training, when performed properly, stimulates the development of lean muscle mass, which means more energy expenditure or higher (faster) metabolism at rest. More lean muscle equals more calories burned during exercise, a good portion of these coming from fat sources, along with an increase in the number of calories that are used during rest.

7. What about strength training for seniors? Is it recommended?

The benefits of resistance exercise for seniors are increased strength, endurance, flexibility, and more energy; though there are some possible negatives such as some discomfort or stiffness—same as in the younger population. Even the sick and elderly can gain benefits that will positively affect their quality of life. The oldest person I personally know of is a 106 year-old man who jogged 6 miles every day and waited tables at the St. Francis Hotel in San Francisco.

Getting more muscle strength will carry over into every day activities and quality of life. It also enhances the cardiovascular endurance capability by placing less stress on the heart and circulatory system as endurance activities are performed (at a significantly lower level of effort).

The key is proper *design* and *progression* of a resistance program in order to achieve maximal benefit—regardless of age.

FACTS & MYTHS ABOUT STRENGTH TRAINING AND WOMEN

Many women seem to think that participating in resistance and strength training will cause their muscles to grow excessively and that as a result they will look less feminine. This is absolutely not true for the average woman and is good news for those women wanting increased strength without increased size.

A woman will not experience increased muscle size because of small increases in muscle mass and decreases in fat (adipose) tissue in the limbs. Since muscle tissue is denser than fat tissue these changes combined result in no overall change unless it is a slight decrease in limb circumference. Another good point here is that firm, toned muscle is more attractive than excessive adipose (fat) tissue.

There is always the possibility that some women will show increases in limb size due to strength training because of several factors:

- A more intense training program than one the average woman would be able to tolerate.
- A genetic factor which can lead to developing greater muscle mass.
- Lower than normal estrogen to testosterone levels.
- Higher than normal testosterone levels.

Comparisons have been made with females and males using identical strength training programs. Results indicate that although a woman's absolute or maximum strength is less than a man's, the difference is virtually nonexistent if it is expressed relative to muscle cross-sectional area, or fat-free mass. A woman's adaptations to resistance training are generally the same or even slightly greater than a man's, which means women do not need to train differently, except that absolute or maximum resistance is usually less.

Resistance training for women can result in many positive changes, including a fit appearance and increased strength and power for daily life and sport activities. As a result, more and more women are becoming involved in resistance training as part of their overall conditioning program today.

Myths vs. Facts

- **Women Can't Get Strong!** - Myth! Fact: It is a fact that women tend to gain strength slightly faster than the average man does.

- **Strength Training Defeminizes Women!** - Myth! Fact: Strength training will make a woman look and feel better about herself. Tight, firm muscles have nothing to do with the term defeminizing.

- **Strength Training Causes Big Muscles!** - Myth! Fact: Most women simply don't have the genetic potential to gain large muscles. The level of testosterone is responsible for the development of muscle bulk and women generally do not have sufficient amounts. Women with large amounts of muscular development as seen in "muscle" magazines didn't get it the old fashioned way, and they undoubtedly had chemical help with either steroids or synthetic derivatives of growth hormone.

- **Women Can Get Muscle-Bound!** - Myth! Fact: The term muscle-bound indicates a lack of flexibility. Strength training done properly actually can enhance flexibility. The key here is using full range of motion during each training exercise.

- **No Pain, No Gain!** - Myth! Fact: I don't know where this got started. A proper training program should not be painful; challenging and uncomfortable maybe, but certainly not painful. I think the "no pain, no gain" concept equals "no sense."

- **Muscles Can Turn To Fat!** - Myth! Fact: Muscles do not have the physiological capability to change into fat. This is absolute nonsense! If a muscle isn't used, it gets smaller (atrophy); in other words: Use It or Lose It!

- **More Is Better!** - Myth! Fact: Sooner or later during training you reach the point of diminishing returns or no return at all. The key is quality training, not quantity training.

- **Protein Supplements Are Essential For Muscular Development** - Myth! Fact: This statement has no scientific basis at all. Protein ingested in excess of your body's needs is not used to build muscle tissue. In fact, if consumed in excess of the body's needs it will be converted to fat and stored. Excessive protein can lead to a loss of urinary calcium and is a concern because of the risks of osteoporosis, especially in women.

- **Proper Strength Training Must Be Complex!** - Myth! Fact: It is really just the opposite. A good "basic" strength-training program gives the best potential for success.

- **Strength Training Can Rid the Body of Fat!** Myth! Fact: Strength training will not totally eliminate fat. Some fat is needed for normal bodily functions and there are two types: **essential fat** and **storage fat**. Essential fat is necessary for various body structures such as the brain, nerve tissue, bone marrow, heart, and cell membranes. Adult women have about 12% of their weight in essential fat. Storage fat represents the excess energy that has been stockpiled. The acceptable level of **total fat** for men should range from 15-17%. The acceptable level is generally considered to be 22-24% for women.

- **Strength Training is for Young People!** Myth! Fact: It is never too late to experience a higher quality of life. Good studies show that older women experience significant health improvements following participation in strength training programs: increases in bone density and muscle mass. It is important though, as with any form of exercise, that you check with your physician before starting a program.
- **Strength Training Can't Be Fun!** Fact: Why not? It should be an enjoyable time in your life and a weekly routine. It is fun watching your body become toned and strong and more flexible.

- **Strength Training Is A Contest!** Myth! Fact: This is ridiculous. Don't compare your numbers to someone else's numbers. Do your very best during a workout and leave it at that.

Important Facts About Minerals for Women

Approximately 4% of your body mass consists of 22 elements called minerals which are distributed in all body tissues and fluids. Minerals occur freely in nature, in soil, and the waters of rivers, lakes, and oceans. The root system of plants absorb minerals from the soil and become incorporated into the tissues of animals that eat plants.

Minerals function primarily in metabolism as constituents of enzymes and also provide structure in the formation of bones and teeth. They also synthesize the biologic macronutrients of glycogen, fat, and protein.

A balanced diet will generally provide adequate mineral intake, except in some geographic locations lacking specific minerals such as iodine.

Osteoporosis has now reached almost epidemic proportions among older individuals, particularly women. But adequate calcium intake and regular weight-bearing exercise and/or resistance training will provide an effective defense against bone loss at any age.

Note here that women who train intensely, but who do not match energy intake to energy output reduce body weight and body fat to the point that may adversely affect menstruation. These women often show advanced bone loss at an early age but it is important to know that restoration of normal menstruation does not totally restore bone mass.

The relationship between muscular strength and bone density supports using strength testing of postmenopausal women as a useful tool to screen for osteoporosis.

About 40% of American women of childbearing age suffer from dietary iron deficiency that could lead to iron-deficiency anemia. This condition will negatively affect aerobic exercise performance and the ability to perform intense training.

Iron deficiency anemia impairs the body's ability to transport oxygen and process it in energy transfer reactions. This can cause general sluggishness, loss of appetite, and reduces the capacity to sustain even mild exercise.

For women on vegetarian-type diets, the relatively low bioavailability of non-heme iron increases the risk for developing iron insufficiency. Both vitamin C (best obtained in food) and moderate exercise increase intestinal absorption of non-heme iron.

Regular exercise will not generally create a significant drain on the body's iron reserves.

CHILDREN AND
STRENGTH TRAINING

Can strength training harm the skeletal system of prepubescent children? Can prepubescent children get stronger during strength training? This is still a controversial topic. I want to stress here that there is a difference between resistance/strength training and weight lifting. Resistive/strength training involves performing exercises in an attempt to make the individual stronger and does not have to involve the use of maximal or near maximal resistance or weights for that matter.

In weight lifting, the primary objective is to lift as much as possible for one repetition, (Olympic and power lifting) thus the need for maximal resistance during training.

Research clearly demonstrates that resistive/strength training can cause significant increases in strength and can be achieved without injury to children in a well-organized and supervised program. The concern about the possibility of acute and chronic injuries to children is a valid one; therefore the training program should NOT focus on lifting maximum or near maximum amounts of resistance. The number of repetitions should be a minimum of 10, with resistance set no greater than a 10-repetition maximum, unless you are using the Isorobic concept.

Children need to develop cardiovascular fitness, flexibility, and motor skills as well as strength. Much of the strength development will come as a result of motor skill training (running, jumping, throwing, etc.). The emphasis should be on safety and enjoyment. Prior to any exercise program, including resistance/strength training, all children should have a medical examination by a physician knowledgeable in sports medicine.

Though it depends on the physical and mental development of the individual child, a general rule is that there should be no maximal lifts until the age of 16 has been reached.

What is Prepubescent? Boys aged 13-14 and girls 11-12. The problem is that prepubescent boys and girls need to be educated about the effects and benefits of proper strength training and learn the difference between weight lifting and strength/resistive training.

Young people need "functional" strength of the overall body. Weight lifting is measured by the amount of weight lifted one time. So if you are not a competitive weight lifter you should not be training like one.

The Fundamentals for Training Children

Children should be taught the following fundamentals of resistive/ strength training:

- **Overload** - the muscles must be overloaded to increase strength and demands must increase from workout to workout. Example: doing 5 perfect push-ups (from knees or with straight body) today and doing 6 perfect ones the next day. Resistance can be increased by adding more repetitions or by working against the clock (such as seeing how many repetitions can be done correctly in 15-30 seconds).

- **Intensity** - begin with a resistance load in which fatigue is reached within a prescribed number of repetitions. Once proper technique is learned, it becomes easier to challenge the child with more resistance and yet maintain safety. As youth develop physically and mentally their intensity can gradually be increased.

- **Double Progression** - if using weights, use a resistance (if possible) that he or she can do 10 repetitions with. This should be done during each workout until 15 repetitions can be done. When this occurs, increase the weight by 5% or less. Progression is done by first increasing repetitions and then by increasing weight (double progression). Pre-pubescents should perform 20-25 repetitions for their hips, 15-20 for their legs and 10-15 for the upper torso.

- **Full Range of Motion** - this is critical! No cheating! This helps maintain flexibility and lowers the potential for injury. Any weight should be lifted in a controlled manner so momentum doesn't have an effect on the exercise. If full range of motion cannot be maintained, the weight is too much and should be lowered until it can.

- **Train 2-3 times per week** - I recommend that youth train two days per week in the beginning on non-consecutive days. The recovery of the muscle is just as important as the exercise itself so more is not necessarily better. Between 48 and 72 hours is usually needed for the body to recover from a workout.

- **Using a split routine, alternating body parts on different days, is NOT recommended** for several reasons:

    1. The body needs 48 hours minimum to recover its energy stores (carbohydrates).
    2. Second, split routines are inefficient in terms of time and a strength program should not be the focal point of a youth's entire week; fun should be the focal point!
    3. Finally, split routines can lead to over-training, producing more wear and tear on a young body.

- **Exercise Largest to Smallest Muscles**- The smaller muscles are used to assist the larger ones in exercise. Since they are smaller you don't want to fatigue them first.

- **About 9-14 Different Exercises Per Workout** - I recommend that beginners start with no more than 9 exercises. The lower volume decreases the potential for injury. He or she can progress to 14 exercises once the initial ones can be performed safely and correctly. Nine muscle groups should be considered: hips, hamstrings, quadriceps, calves, chest, upper back, shoulders, abdominals, and lower back. Target one exercise for each of these 9 areas.

- **Accountability** - Maintain adequate records of performance and progress. Why? It provides immediate feedback on improvement. It is a great motivation tool. Individuals need to feel good about themselves, and they are motivated by achievement.

Should Kids Lift Weights?

I think there are two major requirements:

1. They should be **mentally mature** enough to know why they are training and what they are doing. The ability to concentrate is an important factor in any resistive exercise program.

2. They should be **physically mature**, beyond puberty.

The reasoning that weight training is dangerous for children is still valid. In my opinion prepubescent children should never engage in Olympic or Power lifting and should always have qualified supervision for any kind of weight training. Children can't take the same kind of stress as adults and their bones are still growing.

With the above factors in mind is it possible for young boys and girls to gain strength through training? Of course, but within reason. I think the emphasis should be on overall conditioning and strengthening the ligaments and tendons. Ligaments connect bone to bone and tendons connect muscles to bone; training should concentrate on these areas.

Once again, I have to recommend the Isorobic exercise program because the equipment only weighs two pounds, is portable, can be adjusted from less than one pound, to hundreds of pounds, is easy to use, is inexpensive, and doesn't put undue stress on young, growing joints. You can get information on this program by calling 1-866-204-8786 or checking out my web site at **www.JackMedina.com**. I personally have used this program with children and athletes from 7 years of age to Olympic competitors and have had great success. It is a very safe program.

A Question I Am Often Asked:

What about my abdominal muscles and low back? Is there an exercise, or series of exercises I can do (without equipment) that are good for these areas? The answer is YES!

Before I give you the exercises I recommend I want to re-state something I made reference to earlier in this book: You cannot lay on it, sit on it, shake in it, vibrate in it, get wrapped up in it, or rub it on your body to get in shape! The infomercials you see on television and ads you read about electronic devices you strap around your waist that give you the equivalent of 700 muscle contractions and take inches off your waist are simply not true. If they were, and if there were "fat burners" to go with them, there would be no fat, out of shape people.

I recommend a sequence I call **FOUR ON THE FLOOR**! Drawings of these exercises along with an explanation of each follow. One additional note here: Do you remember doing leg-raises when you were in school? Laying on your back, legs straight, trying to lift them somewhere between 6 and 10 inches at a time; either doing repetitions or holding in this position? Well if you want a bad back this is a wonderful exercise. The muscles in your low back have to shorten in order to compensate for the length of your legs as you try to elevate them, ultimately leading to back problems.

To eliminate this problem, making this exercise safe, lay on your back supported on your elbows as if you are watching a television set that is down near your feet. Now press your low back down to the floor (pelvic tilt). In this position you can lift your legs, making your abdominal muscles do the work instead of your low back. This is what we should have been doing when I was in school to help make our abdominal muscles strong instead of making our backs weaker.

To do the "**Four on the Floor**" exercise sequence you have to be able to lie on the floor. Start by doing each exercise as many times as you can in one minute. You may not be able to do a full minute of each exercise in the beginning—it's okay! The object is to work up to one full minute of each exercise (without stopping) doing one exercise after the other with no rest in-between. Each day do the exercises in a different order. You will find your entire abdominal area getting stronger and flatter, while your low back gets stronger!

Four on the Floor

Floor Curl:
1. Curl forward toward your knees.
2. Keep low back and feet on the floor.
3. Work toward doing one full minute of this exercise.
4. Works middle abdominals and back.

Reverse Curl:
1. Sit as in Figure #1.
2. Move your upper body backward until you begin to lose balance.
3. Return to starting position.
4. Do not hook your feet under anything.
5. Works low abdominals and lower back.

Hip Lift:
1. Lay on back, arms at your sides, palms to the floor.
2. Lift your feet and knees straight upward as shown in Figure #1 (see arrow).
3. Push down with your arms and lift your hips straight up without swinging your knees toward your head.
4. Works low abdominals and lower back.

Hip Roll:
1. Lay on your back with arms out to your sides, palms down.
2. Elevate your legs to a 90 degree angle.
3. Swing your legs right and left as far as possible; make sure your shoulders and hands do not come off the floor.
4. If you have back problems, bend your knees while doing this exercise.
5. Works the low abdominals, low back, and obliques.

MUSCLE SORENESS

Most of us have experienced soreness and stiffness in muscles and joints that have been exercised. There may be temporary soreness persisting for several hours immediately after unaccustomed exercise, or residual soreness, which may appear later and last for 3 to 4 days. For as long as I can remember I have been told that "lactic acid" in the muscles is the cause of muscle soreness. Actually lactic acid is a by-product of anaerobic glycolysis (glycolysis meaning the first stage of glucose, or blood sugar, breakdown within cells which involves a series of chemical reactions) that also serves as a metabolic intermediate that transports energy from muscle to muscle and from muscle to the liver. High levels in the muscle can poison the contracting apparatus and inhibit enzyme activity.

It is important to understand that lactic acid is an energy source, not the cause of soreness itself, and the replenishment of this energy source involves removing the lactic acid that has accumulated during activity from the blood and muscles. Lactic acid buildup within the muscles causes muscular fatigue. If light activity (walking, stretching) is performed after a workout, the accumulated lactic acid is removed more rapidly than if complete rest follows the workout (Hermansen et al., 1976).

When light activity is performed following a workout, game or activity, a portion of the accumulated lactic acid is aerobically metabolized to supply some of the ATP necessary to perform the light activity. Because of this it is recommended that the rest period between sets in resistive/strength training in which lactic acid is accumulated consist of light activity rather than complete rest.

Causes of Soreness

There are four possible causes for soreness:

1. very small tears in the muscle tissue itself,
2. osmotic pressure changes that cause retention of fluid in the surrounding tissues,
3. overstretching and possible tearing of connective tissue and
4. muscle spasms.

The actual precise cause of muscle soreness is still unknown. I have attended many American College of Sports Medicine conferences and listened as scientists brought forth various theories on the subject of muscle soreness. We do know that the degree of soreness or discomfort depends to a large extent on the intensity and duration of effort and the type of exercise performed. It seems that eccentric (contraction that involves lengthening of a contracted muscle) and to some extent isometric contractions tend to cause the greatest post exercise discomfort.

Theories on Soreness

- **Spasm Theory** - because of an unaccustomed workload, muscles will go into a state of spasm. Stretching immediately after exercise in order to delay or prevent soreness supposedly can relieve this. However, it should be noted that post exercise stretching has not consistently been shown to alleviate delayed muscle soreness.

- **Tear Theory** - this proposes that minute tears or ruptures of individual fibers cause delayed soreness. This is usually associated with eccentric contractions which put a greater strain on connective tissue and muscle fibers than does concentric (contraction that involves shortening of the contracted muscle) muscle action.

- **Excess Metabolites** - proposes that prolonged exercise that follows a layoff causes an accumulation of metabolites in the muscle. This in turn triggers osmotic changes in the cell and fluid is retained. The edema (swelling) caused by increased osmotic pressure excites the sensory nerve endings and causes pain. This theory is inadequate to explain soreness because the metabolic stress of concentric work is usually 5-7 times greater than that of eccentric work. As a result, one would expect the metabolite buildup and resulting soreness to be greater in concentric exercise and not in eccentric exercise as is generally reported.

- **Tonic Muscular Spasms** - it is argued that exercise above some minimal level produces a diminished oxygen supply due to inadequate blood flow in the active muscles. This can produce pain and initiate a reflex contraction of the muscle, which sets up repeated cycles of pain, ischemia, and spasm.

- **Connective Tissue Damage** - there is significant experimental evidence to support the argument for muscle tears and connective tissue damage which result in muscle soreness.

It is interesting to note that a single bout of exercise has a significant protective effect on the development of muscle soreness and damage in subsequent exercise. This supports the wisdom of gradual progression when beginning an exercise program.

We don't know exactly what causes muscle soreness. The key seems to be not overdoing it as you embark on your exercise. Take it a little at a time!

FLEXIBILITY

Flexibility is or should be an important part of any training program. I do not recommend that you work on flexibility without warming up first. This might include some walking or light jogging or "slow stretching" as indicated below. It is important to get the blood flowing into the muscles before trying to stretch them.

There are actually four types of stretching techniques and which one you use will depend upon the time you have available, which one you prefer to use and whether or not you have a training partner. As always, check with your physician before embarking on any type of exercise or flexibility program.

Take the Flexibility Test

Here is a quick test to take to check your flexibility:

1. Sit on the floor with your legs stretched out in front of you, knees slightly flexed, toes up. Hold your arms out in front of you (one hand on top of the other), take a big breath and as you exhale, reach as far forward as you can reach toward your toes comfortably (without pain). Don't bounce! Hold for 3 seconds and record the point of furthest reach (middle of shins, to instep, to toes, 1" beyond toes, etc.).

    In my opinion you should be able to outreach your toes by at least 3". If you can't, you are a walking low back-hamstring pull looking for a place to happen.

    Do not do this test in a standing position! When you try this standing, bending forward to check your flexibility, you are working against gravity. You could hurt your back trying to stand up after bending forward. Don't do it! It is much safer to take this test sitting down so you are moving forward and backward, not up and down.

2. Stand with your hands on your hips, index fingers right on the hip bone, thumbs back (fingers pointing forward). You need someone to help you record this measurement using a tape measure. Take a big breath, blow the air out as you squeeze your elbows together as close as you can. Hold this position while someone measures the distance between your elbows (inside elbow to inside elbow). The distance, in my opinion, should be no greater than 10". If greater than this it indicates you have too much stress in the shoulder, trapezius, and neck area. This could ultimately lead to muscle tightness, headaches and nerve pinches which could affect other parts of your body.

NOTE: Once again I have to refer you to the Isorobic Exercise Program which incorporates a great stretching routine into its program. It is easy to do, fast with great results and can be done without a partner and without having to get down on the floor to stretch if it is inconvenient or impossible for you. See page 124 for details.

Types of Stretching

*   **Static Stretching** - this is the most common type and involves a voluntary passive relaxation of the muscle while it is being elongated (see test #1 above). It is easy to learn, effective, and is accompanied by a minimal incidence of soreness or injury.

    Using this technique involves holding the muscle in a static position (no bouncing) at the greatest muscle length possible. There are many variations of this technique involving stretch times up to 60 seconds. Typically a muscle is stretched from 6-10 seconds and is repeated 2-3 times. Each succeeding time you try to stretch further in order to extend the range of movement.

- **Ballistic Stretching** - I don't recommend this one. It involves bouncing or bobbing movements during the stretch and the final stretched position is not held. This type of stretching can lead to increased amounts of muscle soreness and the possibility of injury during the stretching itself.

- **Slow Movement Stretching** - is often used, such as neck rotations, arm, shoulder, trunk, knee, and ankle rotations. This technique is more important as a warm-up activity than it is as a flexibility technique.

- **Proprioceptive Neuromuscular Facilitation (PNF) Technique** - the theory here is that the voluntary contraction of the agonist muscle will provide neural activation resulting in reciprocal inhibition of the antagonistic muscle thus allowing greater range of motion.

What? Using test #1 as an example and using a partner to help you, here is what happens. You try to reach forward (while sitting on the floor or ground) towards your toes as far as you can. Your partner, who is kneeling behind you, tries to push you farther forward while you resist his/her attempts by pushing back against the stretch. This resistance goes on for a period of 10 seconds. At the end of 10 seconds, take a big breath, exhale, relax and let your partner move you forward beyond your original stretch point.

This method can be used with any stretching motion but does require using a partner and takes time to learn correctly. You see improved flexibility almost immediately. However, flexibility, to be maintained, has to be worked on regularly; 2-3 days per week.

The greater your ranges of motion, the less susceptible you will be to injury, providing you have adequate strength to go along with the flexibility.

WHAT IS YOUR BODY MASS INDEX?

According to research scientists, there is a way for you and I to determine whether or not our body weight is normal. It is called Body Mass Index (BMI) and it comes from body mass in relation to stature. However, this will not work for people who are athletes because it fails to consider factors such as bone and muscle mass and even the increased quantity of plasma volume which can come from exercise training. The possibility of misclassifying an athlete as overweight using BMI standards applies mostly to large athletes: shot putters and discus throwers in track and field, bodybuilders, weightlifters, upper weight class wrestlers, professional football players, etc.

But for you and me, our Body Mass Index would be worth knowing; because as your Body Mass Index goes up, so does your risk for cardiovascular complications (including hypertension), diabetes, and renal disease. The lowest risk category occurs for individual's whose BMI's range from 20-25, and the highest risk includes those whose BMI exceeds 40.

BMI Goals

- For **Women, 21.3 to 22.1** is the suggested desirable BMI range. Increases in high blood pressure, diabetes, and coronary heart disease can occur when BMI values exceed **27.3**.

- For **Men, 21.9 to 22.4** is the suggested desirable BMI range. Increases in high blood pressure, diabetes, and coronary heart disease can occur when BMI values exceed **27.8**.

The Surgeon General defines being overweight as a BMI between 25 and 30; a BMI in excess of 30 defines Obesity.

Calculating Personal BMI

So now it is your turn to find out your own BMI. Use the following formula:

- **Step 1.** Multiply your body weight (in pounds) by 0.45 (converting your pounds to kilograms).

- **Step 2.** Multiply your height (in inches) by 0.0254 (converting height to meters).

- **Step 3.** Multiply the answer in step 2 by itself (to obtain square meters).

- **Step 4.** Divide the result of Step 1 by the answer to step 3 (divide weight in kilograms by height in meters).

The result will be your personal Body Mass Index (BMI)

Example: Body weight = 160 pounds (male)
Height 68 inches
0.45 X 160 = 72.0
0.0254 X 68 = 1.72
1.72 X 1.72 = 2.97
72 divided by 2.97 = **24.24 BMI**

Another way to calculate your BMI is to go to the website:

http://www.nhlbisupport.com/bmi/

THE RIGHT APPROACH TO TREATING ATHLETIC INJURIES:

The proper sequence to use for treating injuries is to use the "RICE" method as follows:

RICE - Rest, Ice, Compression, Elevation

1. **Rest** - With any injury, stop doing the activity you were doing when you got injured. With severe injuries, sprains, strains, bursitis, tendonitis or fractures you must rest; let your physician be your guide. With injuries that are not severe, complete rest may not be necessary. Usually within a few days the injured tissues begin to repair themselves and light exercise can help speed recovery by increasing blood flow; bringing nutrients to the injured area and flushing away waste products. Movement will help get an injured muscle functioning again and allow a quicker return to the activity or sport. How much activity or movement? Let your body tell you. If there is pain, stop. If you can tolerate some discomfort the movement will probably help the healing process.

2. **Ice** - if you don't know what to do when an injury occurs, use ice. You cannot make an injury worse using ice but you can make an injury worse by using heat too soon. Ice reduces blood flow to the injured area as well as reducing swelling and should be applied for 10 minutes on and 10 minutes off. If you notice much redness, stop icing for a few minutes. Absolutely NO Heat should be used for 72 hours (3 days) after an injury!

   - **Contrast Bathing** - one really good treatment, after using ice treatment for 3 days is to fill two sinks with water, one ice water and one hot water (not so hot it burns).

Start by putting the injured part (foot, ankle, hand, wrist, elbow) into the hot water for 3-7 minutes. Now put the injured part in the ice water for 3 - 7 minutes. Go hot, cold, hot, cold, hot, cold, and hot! What does this do? The hot water draws blood into the injured tissue. When you put the injured part in the ice water it shuts off the blood flow. When you return to the hot water again it kind of acts like Drano, flushing waste out of the injured area thereby speeding up the healing process.

- I also recommend you keep a **Hydrocolator** handy. You can purchase one at a medical supply store. After 3 days of using ice you can begin using some heat treatments. These pads are usually boiled in hot water, although nowadays you can usually use a microwave oven to heat them up. Once hot enough they create a steam heat. Take the Hydrocolator out of the water or microwave oven with tongs and wrap it in a towel, placing it on the injured area. A deep penetrating moist steam heat is produced that gets down deep into the tissue encouraging deep blood flow and healing. Most good training rooms and physical therapy departments use Hydrocolators for treatments.

3. **Compression** - wrapping the injured part with an elastic bandage (broad rather than narrow) of some kind will help reduce swelling by restricting blood flow. Do not wrap so tight that you restrict all blood flow. If the area turns blue or gets numb, loosen the wrap.

4. **Elevation** - elevating the injured area also helps reduce swelling; try to get the injured area higher than the nearest joint so gravity can help drain away excess fluid.

The Tendon Sheath Tear

One of the best things that has ever happened to me was having Dr. Don Swartz, D.C, D.O, R.P.T. come into my life. Don was a very special person. I considered him to be "The Best" Physical Therapist, and Chiropractic Specialist in the world. Don was blinded in an automobile accident when he was 16 years old. He became a Doctor of Chiropractic (Missouri Institute of Chiropractic) in 1943 and received his certificate of Osteopathy from Still Osteopathic College the same year, doing it all <u>blind</u> at the top of his class. Don became a registered and licensed Physical Therapist in California 1952. His credentials go on and on and I am so proud to say he was my personal friend and mentor.

Don Swartz was a friend of my parents; but when I decided in 1956 to become a coach Don said, "You need to become a trainer too." He took me under his wing and literally everything I know about injury prevention and treatment of injury comes from this man who is still in practice as of this writing. He can see things by touch you can't see under X-ray or MRI.

Don always gave me this advice, which I share with you: **"If it is swollen and there is pain, use ice. If it is stiff and sore, use moist heat. If you don't know what to do, use ice"**. Great advice!

I want to relate a true story to you that could have an effect on how you look at or relate to injury. In 1967 when I was coaching at Homestead High School in Cupertino, California I had an athlete, named Ralph that had been offered a football scholarship to Oregon State University and was also a very good track and field athlete. During the track season of his senior year Ralph damaged his Achilles tendon and was told by medical doctors that his career was over, he wouldn't be able to participate in either football or track anymore. This meant not only losing a football scholarship but also not being able to participate in the track and field championships that were coming up in a week.

Ralph came to me broken hearted and asked if I could do anything. Remember, during those years, there was no such thing as an athletic trainer. I said, let's make a telephone call to Dr. Don Swartz in Hayward, California and find out what he says. I made the call and told Don what had happened and what the medical profession had said about the injury. Don said, "Get him in here as soon as you can." I contacted Ralph's parents to get permission to drive him up to Hayward for an evaluation.

When we got to Dr. Swartz's office Don immediately looked, by touch, at the injured Achilles tendon, and then asked Ralph to rise up on his toes. Ralph tried but couldn't do it because of the pain. Don then sprayed some cold stuff on the tendon and said, "Raise up on your toes now." Ralph did it without pain! Don said, "You didn't tear the tendon, you tore the tendon sheath. When are the track finals you are supposed to run in?" Ralph said "This coming weekend". Don said, "Have a successful competition". We were dumbfounded! To make a long story short, Ralph ran in the Northern California Track Finals that same weekend, was very successful, got his football scholarship to Oregon State University and played four years of University Football.

What happened? What is a "tendon sheath tear"? How could this affect you? Well, have you ever heard someone complain about having tendonitis or tennis elbow? Just maybe it is not tendonitis at all; it might just be a tendon sheath tear.

Another story is important here in order for a greater understanding of what could happen if the injury is diagnosed wrong. In the 80's I was the Fitness Specialist at Los Alamos National Laboratory in Los Alamos, New Mexico. There was a man there, named "Bun" in his 60's, who had been one of the top softball (fast pitch) pitchers in the world for many years. He injured his throwing shoulder and was told he would never throw again.

Having heard about my background in coaching and training he came to my office in the Wellness Center and told me about his shoulder. Bun said, "I have used ice, heat, ultra-sound, hydrocortisone, ultrasound with hydrocortisone, cortisone injections and complete rest— nothing has worked." I said, "Raise your arm up and circle it in a throwing motion!" He tried but couldn't do it because there was too much pain. I asked, "On a pain scale of 1-10 (10 being the greatest pain) what is the pain level?" Bun said "8".

I said, "Here is what I want you to do: I want you to go home and ice down your shoulder until it is so cold it burns; it will take about 10 minutes of icing and your shoulder will go from cold to numb to burn". He said, "I've already done that and it didn't work". I said, "Watch my lips, I want you to go home and ice your shoulder until it burns, then I want you to do the activity that hurts your shoulder (the softball throwing motion). If it hurts less than 8, keep doing the motion for about a minute, then repeat the icing; repeating the sequence of ice and movement three times in a row. If it hurts just the same as now stop the treatment and give me a call in the morning, we will go from there." Bun left my office mumbling under his breath.

The next morning he called me first thing and said, "It's amazing, my arm goes around in a complete circle. What happened?" I said, "You had a torn tendon sheath not a tendonitis (inflammation of the tendon). Keep doing the treatment every day and see what happens." Well, 3 weeks later Bun was back pitching softball again and was a very happy man."

What is a tendon sheath tear? A tendon connects the muscle to the bone. If you tear a muscle, tendon or ligament they elongate. You treat with ice for 72 hours and then can start using heat; cortisone, an anti-inflammatory, which can be used with or without ultrasound if needed. But sometimes you don't actually tear the tendon; you tear a portion of the sheath that binds the tendon together, the "tendon sheath". This sheath, when torn, doesn't get longer it gets shorter. So in essence what you have is a tendon say 2" long, contracting in a casing that is only 1 1/2 inches long. There isn't enough room, so the nerve fires, giving you pain and you stop moving. This will never correct itself unless you can stretch the tendon sheath out again; but you can't because it hurts too much.

By icing the area you are numbing the nerve, deadening the

pain, so when you do the movement the tendon sheath stretches out again. You can't make the injury worse using ice treatment, but if you use heat on a tendon sheath tear, the tendon sheath can become even shorter making things worse, not better.

This technique often works with people who think they have tendonitis in the elbow (tennis elbow). If they attempt to grab a racquet or even shake hands it is very painful. Try this treatment: measure the pain when doing the activity (scale of 1-10), treat with ice and numb the area, do the movement and see if it hurts less. If it hurts less it is the tendon sheath not the tendon itself. Keep repeating on a daily basis until back to normal. This is what happened to both Ralph and Bun in the above stories.

I only learned this because of Dr. Don Swartz and his God-given gift of being able to see by touch. I have shared this treatment with trainers worldwide who had never heard of it before.

A Tribute to Don Swartz

Don has been a friend of the Medina family for as long as I can remember. He was absolutely the best, and I owe much of my career success to him. From the day I met him until his passing on April 18, 2003, he has been my friend, my mentor, and like a father to me. Don was always available to me when I needed him. He will be greatly missed and remain in my mind, thoughts and heart forever! I LOVE YOU DON!!!! Your legend will live forever!

Jack Medina

DRUGS, ERGOGENIC AIDS AND FITNESS

When I speak at schools across the country I ask the students "Why do kids take drugs?" Invariably I get the same response: "Because it will give me a high!" I then tell the kids (with permission of the administration of course), I have one of the most powerful drugs available today with me and will make it available to you after this meeting is over today if you will give me your attention for the duration of this meeting.

But I need to ask you some questions: How many of you have ever laughed? How many of you have ever laughed so hard you actually cried? How many of you have ever laughed so hard you cried and when you finally finished laughing and crying, you have no idea what started you laughing and crying in the first place; so you start all over again?

Natural High

How many of you have ever exercised? How many of you have ever exercised so hard you huffed and puffed? Did you know that during these two things, laughter and exercise, your brain releases a little chemical called an encephalo-endorphin that is up to 500 times more powerful than morphine; GOD given, free of charge; you don't have to worry about where it came from, what it is mixed with, or what it can or will do to the inside of your body. Why do you think at my age I have all this energy? I have endorphins running everywhere and I got them free and you can have them too.

What is interesting about the above is that most of the kids have never been told this before. Sad isn't it?

Drugs in Sports Today

Many male and female athletes at all levels of competition are using drugs (pharmacologic and chemical agents) believing a specific drug positively influences skill, strength, power or endurance. Using drugs for these purposes continues on the upswing among high school and even junior high school athletes. Among older more highly competitive athletes, illegal drug use remains a cancer out of control.

Prior to the 1996 Atlanta Olympic Games, only two sports, women's field hockey and gymnastics remained free from detection of anabolic steroids. This, despite the fact that there is little "hard" scientific evidence indicating a performance-enhancing effect of many of these chemicals. It is amazing to me that athletes usually go to great lengths to train hard, eat well-balanced meals, receive medical attention even for minor injuries—and yet purposely ingest synthetic agents, many of which trigger negative health effects ranging from nausea, hair loss, itching, and nervous irritability, to severe consequences of sterility, liver dysfunction, drug addiction, and even death from liver and blood cancer.

A Bombshell:

I give this information to you because it is so vitally important that you understand what is going on. It comes from Exercise and Sports Nutrition by McArdle and Katch and should be read by every parent and serious athlete:

"One of the largest pharmacological experiments in history has been running for more than three decades, namely the administration of drugs to athletes to enhance performance in many different kinds of sports. Notably, androgenic-anabolic steroids were used with particular success for virilization of adolescent girls and female athletes.

Perhaps the most remarkable aspect of the large and still

ongoing global experiment is its widely accepted clandestine nature. Although the drug experiments involve many thousands of athletes, physicians, scientists, and sports and government officials, and although the success of these programs have been publicized through print, radio and television, the nature of the program and its results largely have been kept inaccessible to direct scientific, medical, or judicially valid investigation.

Since the mid 1970's, the use of androgenic steroids and other hormonal performance-enhancing drugs has been officially banned by sports authorities, and their usage has been controlled through analysis of urine samples taken at the time of competition (i.e., after drug withdrawal, a rather inefficient and insensitive method). In addition, in many countries the use of such drugs in sports has been declared illegal and prosecuted. But these methods have had relatively little impact.

Occasionally, some athletes tested positive and were banned from competition for a period, but these occurrences were generally considered exceptions, and the athletes caught were regarded as "black sheep." The reasons for the secrecy and misinformation of the public are multifold and may include the desire to protect the clean image of international sports for political and mercantile purposes.

Athletes and coaches deny publicly and tenaciously the use of these drugs—not only because of the official ban and the recognition that such use is a violation of the principles of fairness and openness in sports, but also because athletes and sports organizations do not want to acknowledge that their achievements were not "all-natural", (i.e., solely due to individual talent and effort), but instead were drug-dependent. Consequently, deception is basic to doping, and athletes, coaches, physicians, and officials have frequently and emphatically denied any use of androgenic hormones, even before these drugs were officially banned.

The role that scientists and physicians have played in this clandestine system is particularly sad, not only because these professionals actively contribute to worldwide cheating, but also because they violated scientific and medical ethics. Remarkably, only a few of the physicians involved in doping have been held accountable for their misconduct and unethical behavior.

After a period of scientific controversy, it is now clear that androgenic-anabolic hormones are effective in enhancing performance in sports. Moreover, as has been demonstrated through scientific and official court documents, including secret doctoral theses and scientific reports, the positive effects of these and other hormonal drugs on muscle strength, aggressiveness, and performance in elite sports were common knowledge and had been practiced since the early 1960's for male athletes and since 1968 for female athletes. By far the most extensive and detailed documentation of this systematic drug abuse has come from secret government files of one of the most successful sports nations of all time, the German Republic (GDR).

An estimated one to three million athletes (90% of male and 80% of female professional body builders) currently use androgens, often combined with stimulants, diuretics and other drugs believing their use helps training effectiveness. The above information should be an eye opener about international chicanery, secrecy, and illegalities undertaken by a government desperate to win in athletics at all costs for political reasons.

The very scientists responsible for testing athletes for illegal drug use administered antidotes (testosterone ester "bridging therapy") to thwart detection and circumvent doping control. The government-sponsored program required thousands of top pre-adolescent, teenage, and adult male and female athletes to use steroids over many years. It subjected them to unknown risks (without informed consent) that eventually triggered disastrous and irreversible consequences (growth arrest, permanent physical disfiguration, abnormal tissue growth, cancer, fetal malformation during pregnancy, psychological debilitation), including death.

The report you just read pulled no punches. It was a Top Secret file uncovered from the German Democratic Republic."

History

Anabolic steroids for therapeutic use became prominent in the early 1950's to treat patients deficient in natural androgens or with muscle-wasting disease. Other legitimate use of steroids include treatment of osteoporosis and severe breast cancer in women, and to counter the excessive decline in lean body mass and increase in body fat often observed among elderly men.

Anabolic steroids have become a part of the high-technology scene of competitive American sports beginning with the 1995 U.S. weight lifting team's use of Dianabol (modified, synthetic testosterone molecule, methandrostenolone). A new era ushered in the "drugging" of competitive athletes with the formulation of other anabolic steroids.

Steroid Use and Life-Threatening Disease

Concern centers on evidence about possible links between androgen abuse and abnormal liver function. Because the liver almost exclusively metabolizes (processes) androgens, it becomes susceptible to damage from long -term steroid use and toxic excess.

Although patients often take steroids for a longer duration than athletes, some athletes take steroids on and off for years, with dosage exceeding typical therapeutic levels (50 to 200 mg per day versus the usual dosage of 5 to 20 mg per day).

The Internet

Today the Internet is full of companies advertising new forms of "enhancement" drugs that are easy to get without prescriptions. I simply refer you to the section in this book on "Scientifically Evaluating Research Claims". Where is the research to support these claims? In what professional journal has it been published? Where was the research done? Was it third party, double-blind randomized? I think not!

Ergogenic Aids to Know About

Steroids

- What are "anabolic steroids"? They are male sex hormones which have an androgenic or masculating effect.

- Developed by Hitler - he had them made in order to make his bodyguards bigger.

- Dianabol, Androyd, Nilevor, Maxibolen, Winstrol, and Anavar are a few more common ones.

- Many users of Anabolic Steroids take 10-20 times the therapeutic dose.

Effects of the drug:

- Weight gain - usually water retention
- Strength gains

- Androgens are associated with liver dysfunction, liver cancer, infertility, menstrual dysfunction, male baldness, and deepening of the voice in women.

- They can produce a rapid and profound lowering of HDL's; a low level is associated with the incidence of coronary artery disease.

- Steroids increase the sex drive, cause decrease in sperm count and ability to conceive.

- The American College of Sports Medicine states that anabolic steroids do NOT increase aerobic power or capacity for muscular exercise.

- If a non-athlete uses steroids they get flabby.

Considerable literature is available on athletic performance and the benefits of alcohol, amphetamines, epinephrine, aspartates, red cell infusion, caffeine, steroids, protein, phosphates, oxygen rich breathing mixtures, gelatin, lecithin, wheat-germ oil, vitamins, sugar, ionized air, music, hypnosis and even cocaine.

Growth Hormone (L-Dopa):

- Can cause organs to grow uncontrollably

- May replace anabolic steroids

- Also known as Somatotrophic Hormone (STH)

- Stimulates protein synthesis, speeds breakdown of fat

- Decreases carbohydrate utilization by the body

- Obtained from human cadavers (pituitary gland). It takes 50 cadavers to make one dose. Also made from dead animals (pituitary gland) and sold to athletes.

Amphetamines:

Also known as PEP pills - stimulate the central nervous system;

- Benzedrine and Dexedrine are most frequently used.

- Cause rise in blood pressure, pulse rate, cardiac output, breathing rate, metabolism, and blood sugar level.

- Athletes use them in hopes of increasing alertness and capacity to perform work.

- Continual use can lead to physiologic or emotional dependency, headaches, dizziness and confusion.

- No good scientific results have been seen.

Pangamic Acid (vitamin B-15):

- It is purported to increase cellular efficiency in using oxygen, and reduces lactic acid buildup (thus enhancing endurance). This is what the athletes say, not what science says; there appears to be no physiologic basis on which to use this as an aid.

- Is NOT a vitamin but rather Pangamic Acid; a Russian formula. It has no vitamin or pro-vitamin properties, and appears to serve no particular need for the body. It does not make muscles more efficient.

- Synthetic mixtures are sold as vitamin B-15 and may be harmful to the body.

- The Food and Drug Administration states that it is illegal to sell this as a dietary supplement or drug.

- It can cause liver cancer in 7 years.

Recreational Drugs:

Alcohol - impairs performance!

Marijuana - increases blood pressure and inhibits perspiration which can dangerously raise body temperature.

Cocaine - used by athletes to "get up" for games. It has a 7 minute "positive effect time".

Periactin - used by prescription for itching. If overused it can cause an average weight gain of one pound per week (fluid retention).

Alkalies - Athletes think they gain muscle improvement; no scientific evidence supports this.

Ginseng - promotes menstruation and contains 17 hydroxylated steroids.

Octacosanol - it is an alcohol. If combined with Guarana (which is 2.5% to 5% caffeine) it is called "Boost". It has 5-10 times more caffeine than coffee and is sold in health spas and health food stores.

Free Form Amino Acids - a few years ago there was no problem, and they were originally made in Santa Cruz, California. Now they have an egg base and the Nitrogen content is much higher, which can cause kidney damage. It is now considered **very dangerous!**

DMSO - has anti-inflammatory characteristics but can burn you; is sometimes contaminated. It is used as a carrier for hydro-cortisone.

Androstendione:

Found in meat and extracts of some plants and is touted on the internet as "a metabolite that is only one step away from the biosynthesis of testosterone." The National Football League, the National Collegiate Athletic Association, Men's Tennis Association, and the International Olympic Committee (IOC) ban its use because they feel it provides an unfair competitive advantage and may endanger health, similar to anabolic steroids.

Androstendione is an intermediate or precursor hormone between DHEA and testosterone, and aids the liver in synthesizing other biologically active steroid hormones.

There is little scientific evidence to support claims about this supplement's effectiveness or anabolic qualities. It is unfortunate that the FDA does not regulate the use of this substance and it is therefore readily available to the public. Professional athletes often use this supplement and thus negatively influence impressionable youth.

Clenbuterol and other B-2 Anabolic Steroid Substitutes:

A great number of steroid substitutes have appeared on the illicit health food, mail order, and "black market" network. This is the result of random testing for competitive athletes for anabolic steroid use worldwide. One such drug, Clenbuterol (brand names Clenasma,

Monores, Novegan, Prontovent and Spiropent) has become popular because of its so-called tissue building, fat reducing benefits.

Clenbuterol is classified as a B-2 Androgenic Agonist. The problem is that only animal studies have been done on this substance and it has NOT been approved for human use in the USA; it cannot be justified or recommended for use as an ergogenic aid. However, medically supervised use may be beneficial in the future to humans in treating muscle wasting in disease, forced immobilization, and aging.

DHEA (Dehydroepiandrosterone):

The safety and effectiveness of this drug gives concern not only to the medical community, but to sports medicine personnel. The quantity of DHEA produced by the body surpasses all other known steroids and because it occurs naturally, the Food and Drug Administration (FDA) has no control over its distribution or claims regarding its action or effectiveness. The International Olympic Committee (IOC) and the U.S. Olympic Committee have placed DHEA on their banned substance lists at zero tolerance levels.

Researchers know very little about DHEA's relation to health and aging, cellular or molecular mechanisms, possible receptor sites, or its potential for negative side effects. Pharmaceutical companies synthesize DHEA from chemical ingredients or extract it from wild yams. Many researchers consider the current unregulated and unmonitored use of DHEA a disaster waiting to happen.

Amphetamines ("PEP pills"):

These consist of pharmacologic compounds that have powerful stimulating effects on central nervous system function. Athletes most frequently use the amphetamine Benzedrine and Dexedrine. These two hormones trigger increases in blood pressure, pulse rate, cardiac output, breathing rate, metabolism, and blood sugar. The dangers inherent in using amphetamines are:

- Continued use can lead to physiological or emotional drug dependency.

- General side effects including headache, tremulousness, agitation, insomnia, nausea, dizziness, and confusion.

- Larger doses eventually lead to more and more of the drug to achieve the same effect.

- Suppression of the body's normal mechanisms for perceiving and responding to pain, fatigue, or heat stress.

- It can produce weight loss, paranoia, psychosis, repetitive compulsive behavior, and nerve damage.

Caffeine

It remains a controlled/restricted drug in athletic competition. The IOC permits athletes to consume some caffeine as long as its concentration in a urine sample does not exceed a set limit. Athletes should know that 4-7 cups of coffee consumed over 30 minutes significantly raises urine caffeine to levels that would cause disqualification from competition.

It takes about 3-6 hours for blood caffeine concentrations to decrease by one-half as compared to about 10 hours for other stimulants. While the effects of excess caffeine generally pose no significant health risk or cause permanent damage, death from caffeine overdose can occur.

Alcohol

Is classified as a depressant drug. Alcohol is abused more than any other drug in the U.S. by adolescents and adults, both athletes and non-athletes. The stomach absorbs between 15-25% of alcohol ingested while the small intestine rapidly takes up the remainder for distribution throughout the body's water compartments. The liver is the major organ for alcohol metabolism and removes alcohol at a rate of about 10 grams/hour or the equivalent to the alcohol content of one drink.

Finally - 60-70% of athletes get drug information from: health club owners, other athletes, muscle magazines, Playboy magazine and Readers Digest.

Conclusion

What everything comes down to is fueling the cell for maximum performance. Athletes will train hard if they know what they are doing and why they are doing it; however, they have to have the tools for success. A cell in the human body simply cannot perform without the correct nutrients. So fuel the cell with good food, plenty of raw fruits and vegetables and then design the exercise program that trains the correct energy system for your activity or sport. Drugs aren't needed to achieve maximum performance. In fact, I want to leave you with something my Father once told me before his death. He said, "Jack, winning is nice, but it's not necessary; and certainly it's not important enough to cheat for!"

TOOLS FOR
MOTIVATING THE ATHLETE

I have been working with young people in sports for the past 38 years, especially in men's and women's gymnastics. Coaches demand a great deal from their athletes but sometimes demands can actually "destroy" an athlete if the "mood" of the athlete isn't in line with what the coach wants or expects on a given day.

The "MOOD" Chart

Oftentimes I have wanted to "push" a gymnast very hard during a workout only to find them miserable to work with, which leads to friction between coach and athlete. As a result I came up with the "Mood Chart."

- I used a 4' X 8' piece of plywood that was painted white and laminated so it would be easy to write on and looked good.

- Across the top, under where in big letters it said, "Mood Chart", we put down some 28 different moods, contributed by the gymnasts: Tired, Hungry, Happy, Ready to Work, Need to Be Pushed, Depressed, Twittery (want to talk), Don't Want to Be Here, Bad Mood, Angry, Sore, etc. You can probably think of many more yourself.

- Lines were put on the board vertically and horizontally to separate categories and names of athletes.

- Down the left side of the board were the names of the athletes.

When the gymnast came to practice, the first place they were required to go was to the "Mood Chart" where a marking pen was waiting for them. They were to check off what mood or moods they were in when they entered the workout area. My responsibility as Head Coach was to go to this chart before or during warm-ups to check on each gymnast so I could get an idea of what to expect during the training session.

For example, if a gymnast checked "hungry" I could make sure the athlete had a quick energy snack (I used JP+ Gummies®, a Juice Plus+® product) before starting hard work. Have you ever tried to get a good workout, or even think straight, if you are hungry? Using this "Mood Chart" I could react to each gymnast, help solve problems if needed, and could get the most out of every athlete during every workout.

I can remember times when I was really going to push an athlete "hard" during a training session, only to find their mood that day did not lend itself to this type of coaching. I could have made a terrible mistake that day by pushing too hard, ultimately ruining an athlete's day and possibly a future.

In fact, after a week or two of having the chart up, the athletes added the "coaches" names to the chart. The gymnasts wanted to know how we felt each day so they knew what to expect from us.

Many times, when we took a break after tumbling—the first thing we did each day after warm-ups and flexibility work, I would find a gymnast up at the "Mood Chart" changing the mood; oftentimes from "sad" and "depressed" to happy and ready to go to work. Why? Because the "endorphins" began to be released into the bloodstream making the gymnast feel good. Amazing!

I feel this kind of chart has application to every sport with every group of athletes. It takes time to make up the chart, but I have found it very rewarding. The key is for the athletes to understand why the chart is being used as a tool to help the coaches know how to react to an individual during training.

The "WINNING EDGE" Board

As a coach, one of the things I tried to do was motivate my athletes to perform their very best and reward them for it. As a result I developed "The Winning Edge Board", which was located in a prominent location in the gym or locker-room. I will describe how I used it for my gymnasts but the idea can be used for any sport and any age group.

- I used a 4' X 8' sheet of plywood, painted it white and mounted it on a wall. In big letters across the top it said, "The Winning Edge."

- Since this was gymnastics I put each event on the board: Floor Exercise, Uneven Bars, Balance Beam, Vaulting, Still Rings, Pommel Horse, Parallel Bars, Horizontal Bar, and All Around.

- Under each event I put 3 or 4 photographs of some of the best gymnasts, in that event, in the world. These athletes were "Role Model" gymnasts I had great respect for; their work ethic, discipline, attitude, moral character, etc.

We then set a standard for our gymnasts in competition. If they received above a certain score on an event, our gymnasts' picture, name and score replaced one of the pictures on the board. The picture stayed there as long as their event score was equal to or better in each competition than the score that put them on the board originally and our "Team" rules were adhered to.

It was a great motivator for our gymnasts and they really got excited about getting their picture on the "Winning Edge Board."

This idea simply gave me a "Winning Edge" in motivating our athletes. I wanted our athletes to look up to and respect the person who was originally put on the board; the person they were trying to replace. You might consider giving this idea a try.

CHIROPRACTIC, NUTRITION AND SPORTS PERFORMANCE

by Renée M. Grant-Vartabedian, D.C.

In recent years, Chiropractors have become vital members of the training teams for many professional and collegiate athletic teams, as well as individual athletes. For example, a large number of golfers on the professional tours have regular visits with a chiropractor. Many Olympic athletes have a close working relationship with a chiropractor.

Why Chiropractic?

Why? Because chiropractic focuses on the positive; the act of making the body better. This conforms exactly to an athlete's constant effort to make his/her body stronger and more proficient. Chiropractic helps to make the body a healthier and more efficient machine, a body that allows the athlete to maximize athletic performance.

In health care delivery, we are experiencing a shift from disease-oriented, physician-controlled outlook to a wellness, performance and patient-centered perspective. Chiropractic care, with its health-oriented philosophical basis and its non-surgical and drug-free methods, is now one of the most frequently sought health care approaches.

Chiropractic is based on the natural law of homeostasis, stating that any living organism possesses the innate organization/intelligence causing it to always express its greatest potential for health and well-being. This organization can be witnessed in the proper functioning of every tissue, organ, and system of the body. A proper functioning body is one best prepared for optimum athletic performance.

Controlling and monitoring proper function (organization and expression) of every tissue and organ is the primary responsibility of the brain and nervous system. A lack of health or performance will result when the nervous system is impaired or damaged by misalignment and/or malfunction of the spine. Chiropractic helps eliminate spinal problems, allowing the body's organs to work optimally, and combined with appropriate health practices, enhances the athlete's optimum health and performance.

History of Chiropractic

Chiropractic emphasizes preventive/wellness care through management plans seeking to prevent disease, prolong life, promote health and enhance the quality of life. A specific regimen is designed to provide for the patient's well-being and for maintaining the optimum state of health and bodily functions. This type of care has been used for over 100 years, founded by Dr. D.D. Palmer in Davenport, Iowa. While examining the neck of Harvey Lilliard, he discovered a protrusion caused by a misplaced bone. After adjusting the vertebra, Harvey's impaired hearing returned three days later. From this beginning has developed the scientific-based field of chiropractic.

Athletic Performance and Chiropractic

"If Not for Chiropractic, I Would Not Have Won the Gold Medal"

Dan O'Brien, Olympic Decathlon Record Holder & "World's Best Athlete"

If you want to compete at your highest level, chiropractic should be an important part of your training along with your workouts, nutrition and rest.

Dan O'Brien has been quoted, "You obviously can't compete at your fullest if you're not in alignment. It was the holistic idea that I liked about chiropractic. I really think chiropractic is essential in running. If I could put a percentage on it, I think I compete eight to ten percent better from regular chiropractic use, if not more. It is essential for me and my training routine."

Ten percent is a huge amount for an athlete, or anyone for that matter. For Dan O'Brien, it would have been the difference between the gold medal and not even making the team.

Considerable research has been conducted on the effects of chiropractic and different athletic injury rehabilitations. It has been used to treat runner's knee, shoulder impingement syndrome, tennis elbow, and almost every other type of athletic injury. These studies have shown a significant correlation between chiropractic health care and increased athletic performance.

Chiropractic and Athletic Ability

One study began by recruiting athletes with the following criteria. They had to be healthy, currently performing, and never under chiropractic care. Each athlete's level of ability was measured through a series of 11 ability tests measuring agility, balance, speed-reaction time, kinesthetic awareness and muscular power. Each test had been researched and provided validity and reliability ratings.

Half the participants were analyzed and placed on a 12-week program of chiropractic care. All subjects continued to train and practice as usual. After 6 weeks, all were re-evaluated and changes in scores for each group were compared. The increases in performance by each group were measured by the average percentage of change of all 11 tests combined.

The control group, those not receiving chiropractic care showed slight improvement in 8 of 11 tests. By combining the average percentage of change on each test, it was found the control group showed an overall improvement of 4.5%

The subjects receiving chiropractic care showed dramatically different results in their scores. They showed improvement on all 11 tests. And, when tested again after the second 6-week period of care, demonstrated a remarkable 16.7% increase in athletic ability, a net gain of 12% more than those not under chiropractic care.

Think of what a 16% gain means in your favorite activity. For a golfer, it could mean an increase in your average drive from 220 yards to over 255 yards! For the runner, a 7-minute mile might be reduced to less than 6 minutes! Chiropractic clearly can make a difference for casual exercisers all the way to competitive athletes. I have witnessed this with patients in my office and work towards that goal in my treatment plans.

Chiropractic and Reaction Time

A landmark research effort from the New Zealand School of Chiropractic and the University of Auckland, has evaluated the effects chiropractic adjustments may have on reaction times. Two groups were tested to study variations in reaction times; one group received spinal adjustments, while the other group, only receiving a short period of rest, acted as a control group for comparison.

There was a marked improvement for the group that received an adjustment over the group that got nothing but rest. The group that got only a rest period did show an average decrease in reaction time: 58 milliseconds, an 8% faster reaction time. The group that received the chiropractic adjustment showed a decrease in reaction time of 97 milliseconds, representing a 14.8% faster reaction time.

Chiropractic and Athletic Performance

Changes in athletic performance and physiological measures in university baseball players were assessed before, during and after a specific duration of upper cervical chiropractic care. Each athlete's performance was evaluated through assessment of the vertical jump, broad jump specified, standing broad jump, and muscle strength.

Physiological measures including blood pressure, pulse rate, microcirculation (capillary counts), and treadmill stress testing were also evaluated. Twenty-one male baseball players, assigned randomly to either a control or chiropractic (adjustment) group, completed the study. The subjects were required to complete three sessions of athletic ability and physiological tests.

The first session was administered before commencing chiropractic care. The second and third sessions were administered after the initiation of chiropractic care at five and fourteen weeks, respectively. Only those subjects in the adjustment group received chiropractic care.

The results showed significant improvement at fourteen weeks in muscle strength (35.7% vs. 7.7%) and long jump distance (3.6% vs. -1.0%) in the group receiving chiropractic adjustments vs. the control group. Moreover, this same group showed significant improvement in capillary counts at five and fourteen weeks of chiropractic care.

Trends in decreased or increased performance in other physical and physiological measures were accompanied by either moderate or large effect sizes within both the chiropractic group and control group. Evaluation of these trends in the group receiving chiropractic care revealed decreases in resting blood pressure and pulse rate as well as pulse rate following treadmill activity. By comparison, trends in these same measures showed increases within the control group.

Mechanism for Increased Performance After Chiropractic Care

How does chiropractic help in increasing strength in athletic performance? The science of Chiropractic is founded on the premise that a proper nerve supply is essential to controlling and regulating the functioning of the human body. Drs. Dean L. Smith, and Ronald H. Cox in their excellent review article entitled, "Muscular Strength and Chiropractic: Theoretical Mechanisms and Health Implications" outline 3 possible mechanisms:

- Removal of nerve root pressure, reversing compression effects.
- Removal of motion restrictions and restoration of normal joint biomechanics.
- Restoration of appropriate patterns of sensory input by normalization of the internal state of the involved connective tissue; enhancing pliability, and increased range of motion.

More and more research today in the field of chiropractic and sports performance scientifically validates the effectiveness and mechanisms of this highly beneficial care.

The Effects of the Aging Process on the Body

As more and more Americans and those in developed countries are living longer, many feel the effects of aging in terms of decreased flexibility, range of motion, coordination, strength, power, and cardiovascular fitness. Continual activity and training into our later years can slow down and even reverse this process, but it takes 10% longer to get the same training effect for every decade over age 30.

Optimal nutrition is also of vital importance in slowing or reversing this aging process. With proper conditioning and nutrition, we have seen those with a physiological age up to 30 years younger than their chronological age, a seeming fountain of youth. Since what we eat "makes the body", the proper building blocks must be there to continually "remake" our bodies as nutrients are used up and turned over. This affects the structure and integrity of the musculoskeletal system in terms of both function and repair.

Nutrition Tips for Sports and the Active Lifestyle

Although many of the basics of nutrition for athletes have been covered elsewhere in this book, I would like to share some tips from my experience working with athletes. Drinking enough water before, during and after activity has been emphasized, but is worth mentioning again. Eating more complex carbohydrates such as rice, whole grains, and potatoes rather than the simple sugars found in sports drinks is important, especially if they are not going to be burned up in a short period of time. The simple sugars, if not burned quickly, will become stored glycogen or fat.

Nutrient density (the amount of nutrition per calorie or per volume) is vital in rebuilding the structural components of the body and for optimal performance. The Nutripoints Program identifies these foods and athletes do well when they pick the highest-rated foods they like, and incorporate them into their diet (see Chapters Three and Four). A "positive nutrient bank account" can be built up from which the athlete can make withdrawals when needed for high performance.

One thing I often see are people not eating properly, or not eating at all before golfing or another activity that will last for an extended period of time. They skip breakfast, and then quickly run out of energy when their blood sugar drops.

I advise them to try this: if you miss breakfast (or can't eat it due to schedule) eat a small handful of almonds (which contain protein and fat to sustain blood sugar over time) or a balanced sports bar (one with a balance of protein, fat and carbohydrate) with a glass of water before you run out the door or to the activity. This really works and is a great method for the convenience-oriented time-conscious person to maintain blood sugar and energy levels.

Tips for Preventing Injuries

Most athletic injuries could be prevented by following the proper procedures. Also, proper chiropractic care on a preventive and wellness basis can keep the body in alignment so that injuries are less likely to occur. We all know the patients who won't come in on a routine preventive basis and they are the first ones to call on the weekends to say, "Help! I've injured myself and I'm hurting—can you "fix" me?"

Most of us jump right into our sport or exercise without a proper warm-up, but it is so important, especially for a morning activity. The first part of a warm-up should be with general overall body movement as with calisthenics such as light jumping jacks, with mild jogging in place, or brisk walking. These general-type movements should then be followed by more specific stretching of the muscle groups, especially those which have been prone to injury in the past.

The back is particularly prone to injury for many, and the key to prevention is increasing flexibility in the hamstring muscles of the legs, which when too tight, cause a rotation of the pelvis backwards and change the angle of the spine. This causes increased stress on the back, as do weak abdominal muscles, further accentuating the curvature of the back. Strengthening the abdominals, the obliques on the sides of the body, and the trunk muscles can set up a structural strength for the back that will withstand most daily and sport activities. Resistance or weight training (done safely and slowly with proper amount of weight or resistance) proves the best for strengthening these. Our poor posture, and sitting on the couch, or in front of a computer all day sets us up for this unfortunate condition.

Conclusion

As athletes become aware that chiropractic care can improve their performance, prevent injuries, and facilitate the body's natural ability for healing, the chiropractor can become the most important healthcare provider to the athlete. If you can keep the parts of your body functioning at 100% of their potential for the rest of your life, you'll have the best chance for optimum health and performance.

While you must have proper nutrition, rest and exercise, the primary control of body function is the nervous system. Chiropractic can play a vital role in keeping the nervous system working efficiently, as well as maintaining the structural integrity of the body, and thus enhancing athletic performance.

Dr. Renée M. Grant-Vartabedian specializes in Family Wellness & Sports Performance. She holds a Bachelor of Science Degree from Aquinas College and a Doctor of Chiropractic Degree from Palmer College of Chiropractic in Davenport, Iowa.

References

Physical Golf: The Golfer's Guide to Peak Conditioning and Performance, Neil Wolkodoff, Kickpoint Press, Greenwood Village, Colorado, 1997.

Topics in Clinical Chiropractic, Dec., 1996; 3 (4); 32-5, 67-8.

To Your Health: The Magazine of Health & Hope. Stern, I., If Not for Chiropractic, I Would Not Have Won the Gold Medal, Dan O'Brien., May, 2000.

The Journal of Chiropractic Research and Clinical Investigation. Lauro A, Mouch B., Chiropractic effects on athletic ability, 1991; 6(4):84-87.

Journal of Manipulative Physiologic Therapeutics. Kelly DD, Murphy BA, Backhouse DP. Use of a mental rotation reaction time to measure the effects of upper-cervical adjustments on reaction time, May, 2000, 23(4):246-251.

Journal of Vertebral Subluxation Research, Schwartzbauer J, Kolber J, Schwarzbauer M., Hart J., Zhang J., Athletic performance and physiological measures in baseball players following upper cervical Chiropractic care: A pilot study, 1997; 1(4):33–39.

Journal of Vertebral Subluxation Research, Dean L. Smith, D.C.,M.Sc.,1 and Ronald H. Cox, Ph.D., Muscular Strength and Chiropractic: Theoretical Mechanisms and Health Implications, 3(4), 1999-2000.

Today's Chiropractic, Mar./Apr., 1996; 25 (2); 28-31.

CHAPTER THREE

FUELING THE BODY
FOR PEAK PERFORMANCE

THE ULTIMATE MEDICINE:
IT'S CALLED FOOD!

The advancements made in sports nutrition have benefited both athletes and fitness enthusiasts. In fact, sports nutrition is now one of the most heavily researched areas of nutrition.

Commonly, exercise enthusiasts and athletes limit caloric intake in hopes of losing body weight, either for athletic pursuits (wrestling, gymnastics, dance, etc.) or to hopefully look better. The ultimate goal is to reduce body fat and maintain lean mass or even gain lean muscle.

Frequently, poor research or misinterpreted research has provided the fuel for recommendations that are incorrect, unsubstantiated, and even dangerous to health or sports performance.

Nutritional recommendations should be based on the basics of energy intake and expenditure. Caloric intake to maintain body weight depends on your basal metabolic rate and activity level. For example, the person with the greatest amount of lean body mass would have a higher resting energy expenditure (basal metabolic rate).

However, it is not possible to exactly count a calorie, along with the fact that daily nutritional needs may vary based on exercise intensity and other factors such as hormonal levels, especially in females.

For many athletes, including those who seek physique enhancement, weight loss is often the primary goal, especially in sports such as wrestling, boxing, and weightlifting, where in many cases rules dictate weight loss. Also, in sports such as gymnastics and distance running, where there are no weight limitations, low body fat levels are considered optimal for performance. In fact, weight and body fat loss is often the primary objective for anyone pursuing physique improvement. People, including athletes, in pursuit of weight loss, adopt nutritional principals that are ineffective and potentially harmful. For example, drastically reducing caloric intake is not only associated with a reduction in performance, but can cause adverse changes in vitamin and mineral status. Improper rates of weight loss can also encourage a loss of lean body mass and glycogen stores, and increase the likelihood of dehydration.

If it is done correctly, simultaneously losing body fat and gaining lean body mass is possible through proper training and caloric restriction. To counteract the potential for muscular losses and resulting decrease in metabolic rate during caloric restriction, resistance training and an increase in dietary protein should go along with attempts at weight loss. It is important to note that initial weight loss from caloric restriction is mostly water loss, especially within the first 3 days. In fact, as much as 70% of weight loss achieved through reducing calories by 1000 kcal/day can be the result of water loss.

As a general guideline, the ideal rate of weight loss is approximately 1% per week, which can be achieved trough a caloric deficit of 500 to 1000 kcal/day. This is because 3500 kcal equals one pound of fat and weight reduction should not be greater than 0.5 –1.0 kg/wk (about 1-2 lbs.).

The most effective approach to weight loss involves a program that decreases dietary caloric intake and burns calories through exercise. Many studies have shown that adding exercise to a weight loss program results in a greater loss of body fat, while maintaining or increasing lean body mass.

WHAT TO EAT BEFORE, DURING AND AFTER EXERCISE

Energy system function and exercise training success is dependent upon delivering the needed nutritional components to the cell or cells involved. In other words, fueling the cell for maximum performance.

Eating Before Exercise

What you eat before your workout can directly affect your performance. The best food for you in particular will depend on you physically and psychologically—we all have little differences that are unique to us. The best foods can even vary from sport to sport, and there will be some trial and error in finding what is best for you. Let's start by looking at some general guidelines.

The goals you have for what you eat before a workout or competitive event are to:

- Keep your blood sugar (glucose) level high enough to avoid hypoglycemia (low blood sugar) which could cause light-headedness, blurred vision, or fatigue.

- Keep your stomach somewhat full to avoid hunger and absorb some of the gastric juices.

- To directly provide fuel for muscles for the short-term (glucose) and long-term (glycogen) during the session.

- To keep you psychologically alert and at your peak mental sharpness.

Athletes should eat a diet of 60-65% carbohydrate, 12-15% protein and 20-25% fat 2 to 3 hours prior to a competition or hard workout. You want to avoid foods that are rich in fiber, and highly seasoned foods because they can cause intestinal gas. For athletes prone to gastrointestinal distress like nausea, cramps, diarrhea, or indigestion before and/or soon after starting competition or hard workouts a moderate liquid pre-game or post-game meal should be considered. There is no difference between an equal amount of carbohydrate in a liquid or a solid form; it is just sometimes easier to digest in a liquid form.

No foods consumed just prior to a competition will lead to super performance. You want something that will satisfy your hunger and will empty the gastrointestinal tract quickly. This is why sometimes a liquid meal may be beneficial; you get needed fuel without distress in the digestive system and are not hungry just before a competition or workout.

You want to avoid large amounts of sugar in liquid and/or solid form 30 to 45 minutes prior to any exercise, particularly endurance exercise.

- If you exercise in the morning, you will need to intake adequate carbohydrates the evening previous so that glycogen levels are not low by the morning.

- It is also important to intake enough food and carbohydrates for breakfast. Protein is also important to help sustain glucose levels throughout the day and between meals.

- Fat intake should be limited in general, and specifically before workouts.

- Meals should be eaten 1-2 hours (if a light meal) or 2-3 hours (if a larger meal) before the exercise session. If you eat too far ahead, say 4-5 hours before an event, you will be hungry and not perform well in your activity. In this case it would be wise to add a small light meal or snack 1 hour in advance of the activity.

- If you have trouble with food still being digested up until the time of the activity, try a liquid meal such as Juice Plus+ Complete®. It can be mixed with water, fruit juice, milk, or soymilk to get the best results for the particular individual.

- A small amount of carbohydrates can be eaten 5-10 minutes before a workout to boost glucose levels. JP+ Gummies®, a fruit and vegetable-based carbohydrate containing the Juice Plus+® powders would be an excellent source for this purpose.

- Previous to a competitive event, drink extra water the day or night before. It is a good idea to consume 8-16 ounces of water 1 1/2 to 2 hours prior to exercise to promote adequate hydration and allow time for excretion of any excess water, and 5-10 minutes previous to the event.

Eating During Exercise

- In general, you will need to make sure you are eating the right types of foods at regular intervals to maintain muscle glycogen, which is used to produce glucose, or blood sugar, throughout your exercise or competitive event.

- If the exercise session is long, 60-90 minutes or more, a small amount of carbohydrates can be eaten during the session to maintain glucose levels.

- The most important nutrient to consume during exercise is water! Please make note here, during forced dehydration (water loss) as in wrestling, the athlete is not losing body fat, he or she is losing athletic performance!! This can occur in any sport! Athletes should drink small amounts of water as often as possible during training and competition.

Eating After Exercise

- After exercise, immediately replace body fluids with water, juices, watery foods (such as fruits and vegetables), or a high nutrient sports drink.

- Eat a small amount of carbohydrate such as fruit juice 15 minutes after a longer workout or competitive event to begin glycogen build-up and replace lost electrolytes.

- Eat meals including carbohydrates (and low fat proteins to a lesser extent) starting 2 hours after the event to continue the process. This process should start as soon as possible after competition or workouts because the tissues of the body have to begin the repair and replenishing process.

- Water and other fluid intake before, during and after exercise is critical (see "Maintaining the Right Fluid Balance" p. 65). The amount of fluids you need to intake is the amount it takes to get your body weight back to the level just before the workout, or competitive event. If body weight can be maintained by fluid intake during the event, endurance will be extended tremendously.

  Normally our body needs 1/3 more water or fluids than our thirst tells us due to a delay mechanism. Another way to know if you're getting enough fluids is to note the color of your urine. The lighter the color (clear is best), the better hydrated you are.

What Foods to Eat

The recommendations in this section are based on the Nutripoints™ Program for Optimal Nutrition (**www.Nutripoints.com**). Nutripoints rates every food for 26 "positive" and "negative" factors as follows:

ESSENTIALS		EXCESSIVES
Protein	Calcium	Calories
Dietary fiber	Iron	Cholesterol
Vitamin A	Vitamin C	Total fat
Thiamin (B_1)	Riboflavin (B_2)	Saturated fat
Pyridoxine (B_6)	Niacin	Sodium
Potassium	Magnesium	Sugar
Phosphorus	Pantothenic acid	Caffeine
Zinc	Vitamin B_{12}	Alcohol
Complex Carbohydrates	Folic Acid	

The higher the Nutripoint score for a food, the higher its nutritional value. The goal of the Program is to eat **at least** 100 Nutripoints from servings of foods in 6 Nutrigroups:

Vegetables
Fruits
Grains
Milk/Dairy
Legumes/Nuts/Seeds
Meat/Poultry/Fish

Because the athlete needs more food and calories, the Nutripoint goal for the athlete is between 200-400 per day for a higher number of servings. This will be outlined at the end of this chapter. (A listing of over 3000 foods is included in the complete Nutripoints™ Program which is available at **www.Nutripoints.com** or 1-888-796-5229.)

So let's discuss the major components of the athlete's diet and how and where to get them.

Carbohydrates

Blood and muscle sugars are primary sources for the body. Sixty to sixty-five percent of the athlete's diet should come from this source of energy. They may be ingested as complex sugars, such as starch and bread, potatoes, cereals, rice, pasta, beans, nuts, and all vegetables. However, simple carbohydrates, those found in refined sugars such as candy, cakes, puddings, soft drinks, some sports drinks , sugar coated cereals and the like, are terrible for you. Carbohydrates are rich in vitamins and minerals, are low in fat and burn clean in the body, leaving little residue.

Carbohydrates are the major source of fuel for the brain which is very important for the thinking athlete of today. Here again, for athletes requiring a nutritional boost sometime during the day I once again recommend Juice Plus+® capsules and Juice Plus+ Complete® because they outscore (in Nutripoints) everything else in the marketplace. They are simply whole food-based concentrates of high-quality fruits, vegetables and grains, in a capsule, gummy or drink.

Let's get specific now on what this all means and how we incorporate it into our eating plan and day. First, studies show that those with a quality high carbohydrate diet overall perform the best during physical activity. What this means is faster times, more endurance and energy, and less fatigue. The reason is that carbohydrates fuel the muscles directly (see Chapter Two). A high protein or high fat diet will decrease performance and increase fatigue because it takes more work for the body to convert these into carbohydrates to be used for energy. The athlete's diet should be 60-65% carbohydrates by calories. Protein should be 12-15% and fat 20-25%.

Below are listed some of the best high carbohydrate foods based on Nutripoints. The Nutripoint goal is 5 or more points and those listed are much higher, meaning they are high-nutrient performance fuel for the athlete.

High Carbohydrate Fruits	Nutripoints (goal for Fruits: > 5)
12 pc JP+ Gummies® (fruit)	34.0
¼ Cantaloupe	29.0
1 Guava	21.0
½ Papaya	20.5
1 c Strawberries	19.0
¾ c Currants, Black	19.0
½ Mango	17.5
1 Kiwi	17.0
½ c Mandarin Oranges	15.5
1 Banana	14.0
¼ Honeydew Melon	14.0
2 Plums	14.0
1 Orange	13.5
3 Apricots (or 6 pc dried)	13.5
1 Tangerine	13.0
½ Grapefruit	13.0
½ c Blackberries	13.0
½ c Fruit Salad	13.0
½ c Raspberries	12.5
6 oz Orange Juice	11.5
1 Peach	11.0
6 oz Grapefruit Juice	11.0
1 c Watermelon	10.5
½ c Fruit Cocktail	10.0
1 Nectarine	10.0

Fruits and fruit juices are best incorporated in the athlete's diet:

- As part of an overall high carbohydrate diet on a regular basis.
- As a way to increase hydration naturally with high water-content foods.
- As a way to keep glucose levels high just before and during exercise.
- As a way to help re-hydrate after exercise, replenish electrolytes naturally, and begin the glycogen replenishment process.

I would much rather recommend fresh fruits or fruit juice over a "Sports Drink" or "Sports Bar", many of which have a high refined sugar content and have only added vitamins and minerals. Some of the sports bars are high in fat (see Chapter Four). Fruits naturally contain a wide variety of vitamins and minerals, plus hundreds—possibly thousands of phytonutrients (plant nutrients) in a balance which can be more efficiently used by the body.

Fruits are second only to vegetables with the highest Nutripoint ratings of all foods. What this means is that fruits contain a very high ratio of nutrients per calorie. The advantage of fruits over vegetables for the athlete is that fruits have more calories than vegetables and the athlete needs many calories for energy during training, competition, and maintaining their high metabolic rate.

The calories in vegetables are mainly carbohydrates. The problem is, there just aren't that many calories in vegetables to begin with. Therefore, for the athlete to eat enough calories from vegetables would lead to a tremendously high fiber intake, which might lead to gas and bloating. There are some vegetables, however that are higher in calories (such as the potato) or have a high glycemic index (such as carrots) which means the food can be broken down to glucose very quickly for the body to use.

Even though vegetables are low in calories, they are still a superior source of nutrients overall for the athlete. Many of the most beneficial phytonutrients are contained in them, so some of the top Nutripoint-rated choices are listed.

<u>High Nutrient Vegetables</u>	<u>Nutripoints</u> (goal for Vegetables: > 14)
2 c Raw Spinach	75.0
1 c Cooked Spinach	53.5
1 c Raw Broccoli	53.0
2 c Romaine Lettuce	47.5
8 pc Fresh Asparagus	44.0
1 c Raw Cauliflower	40.5
½ c Cooked Brussels Sprouts	40.0
1 c Raw Cabbage	39.5
1 c Cooked Broccoli	38.5
1 c Cooked Cauliflower	37.5
½ c (or 1 whole) Raw Carrots	35.5
1 c Fresh Mushrooms	32.5
8 pc Cooked Asparagus	32.5
½ c Cooked Okra	31.0
1 med Fresh Tomato	30.0
½ c Cooked Carrots	30.0
1 c Raw Radishes	29.0
6 pc JP+ Gummies® (veggie)	29.0
6 oz V-8® Juice	28.5
1 c Cooked Green Beans	24.5
½ c Cooked Mixed Vegetables	22.0
1 Baked Potato	16.0
8 oz V-8® Splash Juice	7.0

One way to increase the calories of vegetables is to "juice" them in a juicer. Thus many servings of vegetables can be concentrated into a small drink—concentrating both nutrients and calories—leading to a high performance food for athletes. Salads of course are the main source for eating these vegetables and should be eaten at least once per day.

Grains are one of the main staples of an athlete's diet. They provide complex carbohydrates and many B-vitamins. The highest quality grains based on Nutripoints are listed. (Foods with * are significantly fortified with added vitamins and minerals).

High Carbohydrate Grains	Nutripoints (goal for Grains: > 5)
1 c Whole Wheat Total® Cereal	64.5*
1 c Total® Corn Flakes Cereal	57.5*
1 c Product 19® Cereal	56.0*
2/3 c Just Right® Cereal	51.0*
½ c All-Bran® Extra Fiber Cereal	43.5*
½ c Total® Raisin Bran Cereal	40.5*
½ c Fiber One® Cereal	31.5*
½ c Nabisco® 100% Bran Cereal	31.0*
1 c Kellogg's® Smart Start Cereal	28.5*
1/3 c All Bran® Cereal	27.0*
1/3 c Kellogg's® Bran Buds Cereal	25.5*
2/3 c Kellogg's® Bran Flakes Cereal	21.0*
1 c Kellogg's® Corn Flakes Cereal	18.0*
1 c Post® Grape Nuts® Flakes Cereal	18.0*
2/3 c Nutri-Grain® Wheat Cereal	15.5*
¾ c Kellogg's® Raisin Bran Cereal	15.5*
¾ c Bran Chex® Cereal	15.5*
½ c Cracklin' Oat Bran Cereal	14.0*
¼ c Grape Nuts® Cereal	13.5*
2/3 c Wheat Chex® Cereal	13.0*
1 ¼ c Cheerios® Cereal	13.0*
¼ c Kretschmer® Wheat Germ	12.0
1 c Wheaties® Cereal	12.0*
1 c Rice Krispies® Cereal	11.5*
1 c Nabisco® Team Flakes® Cereal	11.5*
2 Whole Grain Waffles (Jemima®)	10.5*
1 Low Fat Bran Muffin	10.0
2/3 c Quaker® Life® Cereal	9.5*
1 c Rice Chex® Cereal	9.0*
6 Whole Wheat Crackers	9.0
3 small Whole Wheat Pancakes (Jemima®)	8.5*
½ c Oat Bran Cereal	7.0
2 sl Whole Wheat Bread	6.5
2 sl Seven Grain Bread	6.5
1 Whole Wheat Bagel	6.0
¾ c Shredded Wheat 'n Bran® Cereal	6.0
½ c Wild Rice	5.5

1 c Quaker® Puffed Wheat Cereal	**5.5**
½ c Oatmeal Cereal	**5.5**
6 pc Rykrisp® Crackers	**5.0**
½ Whole Grain (brown) Rice	**4.5**
1 Whole Wheat Tortilla	**4.5**
3 Quaker® Wheat Cakes	**4.5**
3 Quaker® Rye Cakes	**4.5**
½ c Spaghetti	**4.0**

Protein

Essential for life, every cell contains some form of protein. Plants make protein by taking nitrogen out of the soil to make amino acids, the building blocks of protein; there are 20 different ones required by the body. Eight of these (9 in children and stressed older adults) cannot be made by the body and must come from food sources. These are called "essential" amino acids. There are an infinite number of possible proteins based upon the combinations of the 20 amino acids.

Complete Proteins

A complete protein is one that has all the essential amino acids in the right ratio in order to maintain nitrogen balance which allows for tissue growth and repair. An incomplete protein lacks, or is low in one of, the essential amino acids. A variety of foods with incomplete protein can be combined and eaten to provide overall complete protein in the body.

Biologic Value

This term refers to how well the food supplies essential amino acids. High quality protein is mostly from animal sources, whereas vegetable proteins (beans, peas, nuts, cereals, and lentils) are incomplete because one or more of the essential amino acids are low or missing which lowers its biologic value. However, if you eat a wide variety of plant foods (grains, fruits, vegetables, legumes, nuts) all of the amino acids can be obtained because each of these has a different quantity and quality of amino acids.

For example, rice/beans, cereal/milk, or even a peanut butter sandwich contain "complementing" proteins, which provide a complete protein when eaten together. It isn't necessary to eat a balance of the essential amino acids all in one food, meal, or day. The liver stores an "amino acid pool" which it can draw from to make complete proteins when needed.

Getting Our Protein

It is best to eat plant foods to make complete proteins in our body. We can eat animal foods to get complete protein, which the animal has made after eating plant foods. Animals don't have the ability to make a protein and must get it from their food. Although foods from animal sources have complete proteins, a specific amino acid from an animal source is not better than the same amino acid from a vegetable source. The best sources of complete protein are eggs, milk, fish, and poultry. Eggs have the best mixture of essential amino acids and are considered to have the highest quality protein overall (the white of the egg, not the yolk).

The Best Sources for Proteins

Although it would seem convenient to get most of our proteins from animal sources, since they are already complete proteins, there are disadvantages to doing this and advantages in getting the proteins from plant sources. Animal products usually contain cholesterol, saturated fats, and a high consumption is associated with heart disease and cancer rates. Because of their high fat content, this can slow the rate of energy production compared to high-carbohydrate plant sources.

There is also a risk for increased concentration of toxins in the animals from pesticides and contaminants (up to 1000 times greater than in plants). Some people have reactions to the growth hormones in meat which are given to quickly increase the animal's size.

The number of competitive and champion athletes whose diets consist primarily of plant sources and limited dairy products continues to increase. Large amounts of carbohydrate can be supplied to the athlete and others involved in heavy training with a well-balanced vegetarian type diet, while avoiding these negative factors in meat.

Is High-Protein Intake Safe?

Despite its role in nitrogen excretion, there is currently no data in peer-reviewed scientific literature demonstrating that normal kidneys will be damaged by increased demands of protein consumed in quantities above the Recommended Daily Allowance. <u>Muscle mass is not increased by eating high-protein foods despite the beliefs of many trainers, coaches and advertisers. If extra calories are ingested in protein they are either used for energy or are converted to fat and stored.</u> Athletes may need to have a slightly higher protein intake, but this is met by eating more food overall when providing for the increased energy burned during training. Too much protein could put too much strain on the kidneys.

How Much Protein – What Type?

Current data indicates that a dietary protein intake of about 1.0-2.0 g/kg/day (grams per 2.2 pounds of weight per day) should be sufficient for strength athletes. The topic of one type of protein over another is still controversial and until more data becomes available the best advice is to consume a mixture of protein types. An easy way to find your protein requirement is to multiply your body weight in pounds by 0.37. For example, a person weighing 165 pounds times 0.37 = 61 grams of protein.

How does this translate into our daily diet? Here are some examples of protein in foods: 12 oz meat = 72 grams (already in excess of the daily protein needs); 2 eggs = 14 grams, 8 oz milk = 8 grams; ½ cup cottage cheese = 14 grams; ½ cup mixed nuts = 12 grams; ½ cup cooked beans = 12 grams. Vegetarians, including "lacto-ovo" vegetarians who eat no meat and eat egg and dairy products, average 75 grams per day, and the average American diet with meat provides 100-125 grams of protein.

Infants and growing children need more protein; 2.0-4.0 grams per kg (2.2 pounds) of body weight. It is suggested that pregnant women and nursing mothers increase their protein by 20 and 10 grams per day respectively.

About 2-5% of the body's energy requirement comes from the breakdown of protein; but the main role of protein is in the tissue-building process.

All cells are composed of some form of protein. About 12-15% of body mass is protein. A brain cell is about 10% protein, while muscle cells and red blood cells may contain as much as 20% of their total weight as protein. Protein content of skeletal muscle (65% of the body's total protein) can be increased significantly through resistive exercise training.

Loss of glycogen reserves, muscle tissue and protein deficiency are the result of starvation diets or diets with reduced carbohydrates.

Weightlifters, body builders and power athletes, both male and female, often eat up to four times the recommended daily allowance for protein, mostly in the form of liquids, powders and pills. Promoters of this will tell you the body absorbs amino acids faster to enhance muscle growth or to improve strength, power and energy. However, this does not occur and is not supported by well-designed research studies.

A male athlete can expect about a 30% increase in body mass from heavy resistance training over one year. For women, this gain could be as high as 50-75%, probably due to a woman's smaller initial amount of lean body mass. Individual gains are affected by genetics, age and training factors.

Evidence is accumulating suggesting that the availability of amino acids and carbohydrate immediately after the exercise period may be significant in resulting muscle growth.

Whey Protein

Is an excellent source of protein because of its high biological value and amino acid composition with different food properties for nutritional, biological and functional applications. It is a derivative of milk production with an amino acid profile closely related to the amino acids required by the human body and is easy to digest.

Casein

Is also a derivative of milk production and has some unique biological properties. It is easy to digest and provides the body with essential amino acids. Many protein supplements use caseinates because of the high quality of protein; they are low in fat and cholesterol and can contain different amounts of sodium and/or calcium depending upon the form used.

Both whey and casein protein are high quality and supply all of the essential amino acids in adequate proportions for the body.

Egg Protein

Is a very high-quality protein source and is the standard by which other proteins are measured. When compared to whey and casein, egg protein is higher in sodium. If an athlete is sodium sensitive, too many egg whites may not be the best protein source. However, it is a great source of essential amino acids that will serve as building blocks for damaged muscle fiber.

Soy Protein

Soy proteins are high in quality, are free from cholesterol and very low in saturated fat. Soy protein is a quality equivalent to both casein and various animal proteins and contains high amounts of glutamine and arginine.

What soy is lacking are the sulfur-containing amino acids, particularly methionine and cysteine. However, research shows that well-processed soy protein isolates and soy-protein concentrates are essentially equivalent to those of animal proteins. It also shows that soy protein is beneficial because of its antioxidant and immune-enhancing properties.

Protein-Carbohydrate Supplements

Significant advancements have been made in the development of nutrient-dense, protein-carbohydrate supplements. For athletes who need to increase caloric intake, these supplements are a more balanced approach than non-fortified concentrated carbohydrate drinks. Research indicates that ingesting these types of supplements during training may be more effective than simply adding carbohydrate to the diet.

How much do I need? Well, take your weight and divide it by 2.2 converting your pounds to kilograms. Now multiply by .8 for a sedentary person, 1.2 to 1.4 for endurance athletes, or 1.8 for athletes involved with serious weight training, to get the total grams of protein needed each day (depending upon your activity level).

Athletes should get between 12-15% of their calories from good-quality protein. Taking in more than this has not been shown to enhance performance. In fact, part of any excess will contribute to weight gain, while the rest is excreted in the urine.

Both resistive exercise and nutrition provide independent stimulus for muscle protein synthesis and muscle growth. Taking in protein before exercise is more effective than after. In addition, having solid or liquid carbohydrate energy during long-duration practice or competition will help reduce fatigue, increase work output, and improve mood and decision making. Carbohydrate also helps to maintain the function of the immune system. I'm not talking about expensive supplements here. The correct sports drink or energy bar (see Nutripoints lists) can provide this benefit. The carbohydrate provides energy to the muscles and nervous system, including the brain.

The important point here is that you can easily get enough protein during normal meals. If you take in more protein than you need, usually with two good meals each day, the excess is excreted or is converted to glucose (blood sugar), glycogen or fat. If an athlete trains hard it is obvious that more protein is needed; but he or she will need to eat more because they will be getting hungry more often, and therefore will be eating more foods containing the necessary protein. Extra protein, regardless of what you are told, is not required for heavy resistive or other types of exercise. Protein isn't even used for this purpose. Carbohydrate and phosphocreatine are the main sources of energy here. Extra protein will not promote extra muscular growth! In fact, in order to have the potential to gain one pound of muscle in 7 days you must consume 2500 calories more per week than needed, and have a proper resistive exercise program to go with it. And even then you only have the potential; every athlete doing this will not gain a pound of muscle every 7 days. Some athletes gain muscle bulk and weight and some don't. Protein provides the amino acid building blocks to build and repair tissue and synthesize enzymes and hormones.

Wrestlers, because of caloric restrictions, need to eat protein dense foods. No more than 12-15% of athletes or anyone else's diet needs to come from protein. Meats are high in essential amino acids and are a good source of protein, so are eggs and milk. However, vegetarians can certainly get plenty of good nutrition by simply combining the plants properly.

During training and competition, <u>low-fat</u> proteins are important because they will settle well in your stomach and will help keep blood sugar elevated over time to prevent you from feeling hungry and running low on glucose for energy. Some high-nutrient quality proteins are listed below:

<u>Low Fat Proteins</u>	<u>Nutripoints</u> (goal for Proteins: > 5)
1 c Juice Plus+ Complete® Drink	31.0*
1 c MET-Rx® Total Nutrition Milk Drink	23.0*
1 c ZonePerfect Shake Mix	22.5*
1 c Myoplex® Milk Drink	21.0*
2 c Fresh Bean Sprouts (mung)	18.0
½ c Egg Beaters® Egg Substitute	17.5*
1 c Smart Fuel Protein Anytime Mix	17.5*
1 c Cooked Peas (from frozen)	14.0
1 ½ c Minestrone Soup	14.0
1 c Cooked Navy Beans	13.5
1 c Lentil Soup	13.5
1 c Atkins Ready to Drink Shakes	13.5
1 c Health Source® Soy Protein Drink	12.5
½ c Health Valley® Vegetarian Chili	11.5
1 c Nonfat Yogurt	10.5
½ c Split Pea soup	10.0
¾ c Cooked Lima Beans	9.5
1 c Skim Milk or Buttermilk	9.5
1 c Cooked Black-eyed Peas	9.0

1 Vegetarian Burger	8.5
½ c Cooked Kidney Beans	8.5
4 oz Broiled Venison	8.5
1 c Cooked Lentils	8.0
½ c Cooked Garbanzo Beans	8.0
½ c Tuna, Canned/water	8.0
1 c Lowfat (2%) Milk	7.5
1 c Soy Milk	7.5
6 oz Baked Pike	6.5
6 oz Baked Red Snapper	6.5
6 oz Baked Swordfish	6.5
2 sl Vegetarian Turkey Slices	6.5
4 oz Turkey Store Fresh Turkey	6.5
4 Egg Whites	6.0
4 oz Baked Quail w/o Skin	6.0
6 oz Baked Sole	6.0
3 oz Baked Salmon	5.5
2 sl Vegetarian Chicken Slices	5.5
3 oz Baked Trout	5.0
1 Vegetarian Hot Dog	5.0
½ c Tofu	5.0
½ c Soybean Nuts	5.0
½ c Bean Chili	5.0
½ c Lowfat Cottage Cheese	4.5
¼ c Sunflower Seeds	4.5
3 oz Baked Lt Meat Turkey w/o Skin	4.5
1 Bean Burrito	4.0
3 oz Baked Chicken Breast w/o Skin	4.0
3 oz Broiled Lean Beef Round Steak	4.0
3 oz Broiled Lean Beef Flank Steak	4.0
3 oz Broiled Lean Beef Top Loin	4.0
¼ c Healthy Trail Mix	4.0
¼ c Pumpkin/Squash Seeds	2.5
¼ c Unsalted Peanuts (high fat)	1.5

Of course many of the foods listed in all of the categories above will need to be incorporated into your favorite recipes. Some of them may be palatable to eat in their natural form as listed.

Below is a sample day, listing the servings from each group and how they could be distributed through the day and around workouts. The serving size depends on the particular food in each food group as listed in the previous charts.

Pre-Workout Morning Snack (150-200 calories)

1 Carbohydrate (Grain or Fruit) serving
1 Low Fat Protein serving

Post-Workout Breakfast (400-600 calories)

2-3 Grain servings
1-2 Fruit servings
1-2 Protein servings

Lunch (400-800 calories)

1-2 Grain servings
1-2 Fruit servings
1-2 Protein servings
2-3 Vegetable servings

Pre-Workout Light Dinner (400-600 calories)

1-2 Grain servings
1-2 Fruit servings
1-2 Protein servings
2-3 Vegetable servings

Post-Workout Evening Snack (150-200 calories)

1 Carbohydrate (Grain or Fruit) serving
1 Low Fat Protein serving

If there is a workout in the morning and not in the evening, then the evening Dinner and Snack could be combined. If there was an evening workout and no morning one, the Morning Snack and Breakfast could be combined. If there were 2 workouts per day, the eating plan could be used unchanged as given above.

For more active individuals, the number of servings can be increased proportionately to all food groups. The total calories for the servings in this sample are 1500-2400.

Here is how it could look with some high-Nutripoint food choices for the servings needed in each category:

Pre-Workout Morning Snack (150-200 calories)   Nutripoints

1 c Orange Juice (to mix with drink)	**15.0**
1 c Juice Plus+ Complete® Drink	**31.0**

Post-Workout Breakfast (400-600 calories)

2 c Corn Total® Cereal	**115.0**
1 Whole Banana	**15.0**
1 c Low Fat (2%) Milk	**7.5**
2 Juice Plus+® Orchard Blend (fruit) Capsules	**A+ Grade**

Lunch (400-800 calories)

2 Slices Whole Wheat Bread	**6.5**
3 oz Turkey Slices or Veggie Burger	**6.5**
¼ Fresh Cantaloupe and Mixed Fruit Salad	**53.0**
2 c Fresh Spinach, Mixed Lettuce, and Veg. Salad	**105.0**

Pre-Workout Light Dinner (400-600 calories)

1 Cracked Wheat Dinner Roll	**6.0**
8 oz Cranberry Juice	**9.0**

6 oz Baked Fish of Choice	**6.5**
1 Small Baked Potato w/low fat toppings	**16.0**
½ c Steamed Mixed Vegetables	**44.0**
2 Juice Plus+® Garden Blend (vegetable) Capsules	**A+ Grade**

Post-Workout Evening Snack (150-200 calories)

1 Small Handful JP+ Gummies®	**63.0**
1 Small Handful of Healthy Trail Mix	**4.0**

TOTAL 503.0

You can see by the high Nutripoint Score of 503 (compared to the goal of 100 or more for the average person) the athlete or active person eats more food and can get more nutrition in the process—as long as the food choices are healthy ones as in the example. There are many possibilities and food combinations for the day. Your goal is to pick the highest rated foods you like and work well with your body in developing your program. You will be getting optimal nutrition when combining these foods with the high-quality whole food-based concentrates of Juice Plus+®

CHAPTER FOUR

WHOLE-FOOD NUTRITION FOR PEAK PERFORMANCE

Optimal nutrition is important for everyone, and especially for athletes and active individuals. The body is subjected to higher levels of activity and performance, which increases the need for a more perfect balance and plentiful supply of nutrients. Where should this added nutrition come from—foods or a nutritional supplement? We know that athletes need more calories—thus they eat more food. That additional food contains more nutrients for the body. So naturally, to some degree, the additional nutrient needs would be met automatically.

The tendency for athletes when eating more food, however, is often to choose foods that are a little lower on the quality scale just to get the calories they need. Another problem is that no matter how well we eat, none of us are perfect—nor are the foods we eat today. Thus many active people and people in general, are interested in using supplements to their diet for added protection.

But first we must understand that pills can never be a substitute for foods! Nutripoints helps you know what are the best foods for the human body overall. These are the foods which have the highest levels of vitamins, minerals, fiber, enzymes, and phytochemicals. They also contain unknown ingredients with benefits which have not been identified as yet. We also need calories, carbohydrates, proteins, and fats. All of these must come from foods in their most natural, unprocessed state as possible. <u>So this is number one—get the most nutrients you can from eating good food!</u>

OPTIMAL NUTRITION FOR ATHLETES:
To Supplement or not to Supplement?

Even though an athlete is using Nutripoints and has a high level of nutrition, they should consider proper supplementation to help them reach OPTIMAL nutrition for peak performance and health for the following reasons:

- Even though you may be eating a healthy diet, <u>nobody is perfect,</u> and so for whatever reason, we may not get what is best for us <u>every day</u>.

- Even though we eat high quality foods, we may not get the <u>variety of foods</u> we need. Most people eat only <u>20-30 foods or less</u> on a regular basis. Many foods may be out of season in certain regions as well.

- Even if we were <u>perfect,</u> and ate all the right foods and in the right variety, the nutrition that should be in the foods <u>may not all be there</u> due to: growing techniques, depleted soils, transportation losses, or storage, cooking, and preparation losses. Genetic engineering of foods also puts into question nutrient content.

Therefore, to achieve the highest level of nutrition possible, athletes should supplement their diet to "bridge the gap" between their "improved diet" with Nutripoints and an "optimal nutritional intake". The chart below illustrates that before we make improvements in our diets, we reach a certain level of nutritional intake (column 1) well below optimal nutrition.

Using Nutripoints to improve our diet increases our nutritional intake substantially (column 2), but can still leave a gap between optimal nutrition. Adding a food supplement bridges the gap between our best efforts and optimal nutrition (column 3).

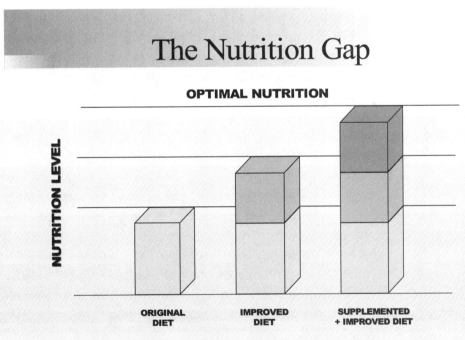

Copyright 2000 *Vartabedian & Associates*

Vitamin and Mineral Supplements: Old Technology

So how do we bridge the gap? What are the best supplements? Until recently, scientists believed that since research studies showed lower rates of cancer, heart disease, and other chronic diseases in populations with high levels of antioxidants in their bloodstream such as vitamins A, C, and E, that supplements containing these nutrients would provide similar results. While studies did show benefits in some instances, one of the startling findings in a major study supplementing beta-carotene (a form of vitamin A) was that beta-carotene in its isolated form did not provide the same benefit as it did when it was eaten in foods; in fact it could be harmful.

The reason, it turns out, is that beta-carotene is only one of many "carotinoids" in the body, so others such as alpha-carotene and lutein are needed as well, and increasing this one carotinoid (which is only 12% of all carotinoids in the body) could throw off the body's natural balance. Since most of the studies showing benefits of beta-carotene in the diet were taken from whole foods, not supplements, this all began to make sense. Even more recently, new studies show questionable benefits and even possible harm from taking too high a dosage of vitamin C in its isolated form out of the context of foods.

We know that there are dozens of mineral interactions in the body, so that if you add one mineral, it can throw off the absorption of another mineral. It could either enhance it, or make it difficult to absorb the other mineral, depending on the amount.

Thus, supplementing with vitamins and minerals, rather than getting them from whole foods can be tricky because their balance in foods is virtually impossible to duplicate, and they may need to interact with unknown factors to achieve maximum results.

NUTRITIONAL BREAKTHROUGH:
"Whole Food" based Supplements

So we can see how traditional vitamin and mineral supplements can pose problems with our overall health and actually cause harm in some cases. This is mainly due to their "isolated" form without their natural balance as found in foods. But what if we could get all of the essence of foods in their natural balance into a supplement? Recently, a new nutritional technology has made it possible to get a "whole food-based concentrate" in a capsule. The concept is to take the juice from a whole high-quality food such as a fruit or vegetable, remove the water, calories, sugar, and sodium, while retaining as much of the original nutrition as possible, and put it in pill form. Thus, you have the nutrient "essence" of the food, and in a convenient form. Since every food has not only vitamins and minerals, but enzymes, fibers, and thousands of recently discovered "phytochemicals"—plant micronutrients with a positive effect but no name or previously discovered benefit, this concept is dramatically superior to taking isolated vitamins and minerals.

The "natural balance" of complementary nutrients in these new supplements enhances the body's absorption for our optimal benefit. Nutrients in whole food-based concentrates are therefore more "bioavailable" to the body, and that's why they are superior and will provide greater protection against cellular oxidation, chronic diseases, and aging.

In the following table the Nutripoint Grades are given for the types and classes of supplements from highest to lowest. The best is this new category, a supplement which is a "whole food" based concentrate. These are basically derived from whole foods in their dehydrated form to supplement our diets to reach optimal nutrition for health and peak performance.

The other supplements with lower grades lack in either variety, completeness, balance, or they contain unrecognized or even harmful ingredients.

The following are the grades for supplements containing:

A+
- A whole food-based concentrate
- Containing a wide variety of high Nutripoint-rated vegetables, fruits, grains, legumes
- Containing natural spectrum and balance of vitamins, minerals, and phytonutrients
- Provide independent scientific research on product documenting positive health benefits.

A-
- A whole food-based concentrate
- Containing only one or a few high Nutripoint-rated vegetables or fruits
- Containing some added vitamins and minerals.

B
- Vitamin/mineral supplement
- Containing a wide variety of nutrients (at least 15-20)
- With approximately 100% of Recommended Daily Values.

C
- Vitamin/mineral supplement
- Which is incomplete (i.e.: 5-10 nutrients)
- Which is imbalanced (i.e. 25% to 3,000+% of RDV's).

D
- Vitamin/mineral supplement
- Which is incomplete (i.e.: 5-10 nutrients)
- Contains unrecognized nutrients (no researched benefits).

E
- Vitamin/mineral supplement
- Which may also contain harmful ingredients such as alcohol, arsenic, aluminum, etc., or harmful levels of nutrients.

Juice Plus+® Capsules produced by NSA, Inc. meet all of the Nutripoint analysis requirements to rate an "A+" as a superior nutritional supplement. The capsules contain a true whole food-based concentrate of 17 fruits, vegetables, and grains with a natural balance of vitamins, minerals, and phytonutrients. They have been independently researched with studies in humans documenting benefits in the areas of: increased blood antioxidant and folate levels, improved markers of immune function, protection of DNA integrity in blood lymphocytes, decreased blood homocysteine levels, and maintaining normal vasoactivity after a high-fat meal.

Antioxidants vs. Free Radicals

The concept of "antioxidants" and "free radicals" seems to be a confusing one for many people. Here is a way to make this idea simple and understandable.

Think of each of the trillions of the GOOD cells in your body being represented by a little round chocolate uncoated candy. You have many different kinds of cells in your body: muscle cells, heart cells, blood cells, etc.

Then there are the "free radicals", the BAD guys that run around in your body too. Unfortunately, these free radicals just love "little round uncoated candy,"(damaged molecules with one electron missing) and at every opportunity they try to take a bite (steal an electron) thus making it weaker or unstable. Eventually this little cell is too weak and can be taken over by the free radical, becoming a diseased cell. This creates a domino effect as more and more weak unprotected cells are attacked

The good news is that "antioxidants" are available to you through good food, particularly fruits, vegetables, grains and legumes. These antioxidants form a shell around the cells of your body (giving each cell a protective "helmet"). When the "free radical" comes along and tries to take a bite it simply bounces off and goes looking for another weak unprotected cell.

This "antioxidant" system is what protects you from disease. So build up your immune system, protect the cells in your body from attack, by eating 9-13 servings of fresh-raw fruits, vegetables, grains and legumes every day.

If you can't do it by eating the right food, you should consider taking Juice Plus+®, which research has shown to dramatically increase the antioxidant effect in our bloodstream and cells.

In the Pre-workout and Post-workout Nutritional Program I specifically recommend Juice Plus+® Capsules as part of the regime due to its high Nutripoint Grade for supplements. A further Nutripoint Analysis shows the following scores for the ingredients of Juice Plus+®:

ORCHARD BLEND CAPSULES		*GARDEN BLEND CAPSULES*	
Papaya	20.5	Spinach	75.0
Acerola Cherry	16.0	Parsley	54.5
Orange	13.5	Broccoli	53.0
Peach	11.0	Kale	49.0
Cranberry	10.0	Cabbage	39.0
Pineapple	8.0	Carrots	35.5
Apple	4.5	Tomato	30.0
		Beets	14.0
		Rice Bran	9.0
		Oat Bran	9.0

The juice powder of a blend of the above fruits, vegetables, and grains listed are contained in 2 capsules of each Blend (the daily recommended serving). You can see that the fruits, vegetables, and grains in Juice Plus+® score very high in comparison to the averages and recommendations of Nutripoints. Remember that the higher the Nutripoint score, the higher the quality of the food (see **www.Nutripoints.com**).

The recommended Nutripoint score for a fruit serving is 5, for vegetables it's 14, and it's 5 for grains. The fruits in Juice Plus+® range from 1-4 times the recommended Nutripoint score (4.5 to 20.5), the vegetables from 1-5 times the recommended score (14 to 75), and the grains nearly 2 times the recommended score (9.0). So this supplement not only is a whole food-based product made from fruits, vegetables, and grains, but from *high quality* ones based on the Nutripoint analysis.

High Protein Drinks for Athletes

Another popular supplement athletes use for their diet are high protein drinks. Some are popular for weight loss, some for a quick meal, and yet others for "building muscles". We discuss protein needs for athletes in Chapter Three, but I did a Nutripoint analysis on some of the popular high protein/milk/diet drinks for comparison. The results are as follows:

Juice Plus+ Complete®, All flavors	**31.0**
MET-Rx® Total Nutrition Drink	**22.5**
ZonePerfect® Shake Mix	**22.5**
Smart Fuel® Protein Anytime Mix	**17.5**
Slim-Fast® Optima®	**16.0**
Atkins® Ready to Drink Shakes	**13.5**
Nestlé's® Sweet Success	**13.0**
Slim Fast®	**13.0**
Soy Protein, Health Source®	**12.5**
Ultra Slim Fast®	**11.0**
Boost®	**8.5**
Carnation® Instant Breakfast	**8.0**
Ensure® w/Fiber	**8.0**
Ensure® Light	**8.0**
Ensure®	**8.0**
Resource®	**7.0**
Resource® Plus	**6.5**
Ensure® High Protein	**6.5**
NutraStart®	**5.5**
Sustical® High Protein	**5.5**
Ensure® Plus	**5.0**
Nutrament®	**4.5**
Sustical® Plus	**4.5**

Most of the drinks with the *lower* scores are high in sugar and fat, and low in fiber. They are mostly milk-based. Those with the *higher* scores are lower in sugar and fat, and higher in fiber. They are mostly soy-based, which is healthier overall. Juice Plus+ Complete® is soy-based as far as the protein source, and contains the Juice Plus+® fruit, vegetable, and grain powders which provide additional nutrients and phytochemicals, thus the highest rating on this chart. Juice Plus+ Complete® is the recommendation here for the most natural nutrition for the athlete desiring a quick, easily digested meal high in both carbohydrates and protein. It could be mixed with skim or low-fat milk, soy milk, orange juice or water. Details on its use pre- and post-exercise are discussed in Chapter Three.

Sports Drinks

As discussed earlier, most of these drinks are very diluted with water but contain a high amount of refined sugar and little or no nutrients. A listing of some of the more popular sports drinks and gels their Nutripoint score is below. Much better in my opinion, would be to use 100% fruit juice to quench thirst and replace electrolytes. To cut down on fruit sugar you could dilute the juice by 25-50% with water.

Ultima® Replenisher	**16.0**
Zing®	**13.5**
AminoVital® Fast Charge Sports Powder	**8.5**
GU® Energy Gel	**5.5**
Accelerade® Sports Gel	**4.5**
Body Fuel®	**4.0**
Cytomax® Energy and Recovery Drink	**3.5**
LowOz®	**3.0**
Gatorade® Energy Drink	**2.5**
Accelerade® Powder Mix	**2.0**
AminoVital® Ready-to-Drink	**1.5**
Exceed®	**1.0**
Recharge®	**1.0**
Endurox®	**0.5**
Power Bar® Sports Gel	**-1.5**

All Sport®	**-2.0**
Lucozade®	**-2.0**
Power Bar® **Recovery Drink**	**-3.0**
Powerade®	**-3.0**
Accelerade® **Ready-to-Drink**	**-4.0**
Gatorade® **Endurance Hydration Formula**	**-5.5**
Gatorade®	**-6.5**

Snack/Energy Bars

Another popular trend among athletes and active individuals is the use of snack bars for energy before, during or after a workout or competitive event. The use of these bars and recommendations are given in Chapter Three. A complete listing of popular snack/health bars and their Nutripoint scores are as follows:

DrSoy® **Protein Bar**	**34.5**
Pounds Off® **Bar**	**29.5**
Clif Luna® **Bar**	**28.5**
Pure Protein®	**25.5**
Tiger's® **Sports Bar**	**25.0**
Snickers® **Marathon**	**23.5**
Energia®	**23.0**
Power Bar®**, all flavors**	**22.5**
Power Bar Pria®	**21.0**
Power Bar Protein Plus®**, all flavors**	**19.5**
Barbell® **Energy Bar**	**18.5**
Power Bar Pria Carb Select®	**16.5**
Bio-X® **Bar**	**15.0**
ZonePerfect	**14.5**
PR Nutrition® **Bar**	**14.0**
Breakthrough® **Honey Graham**	**13.0**
Glucerna® **Meal Bar**	**12.5**
MetaForm®	**10.0**
Atkins Advantage® **Bar**	**9.5**

Tiger's Milk®	9.0
VO2 MAX	9.0
Balance® Bar 40-30-30	8.5
Clif ZBar®	8.5
Slim-Fast Optima® Meal Bar	8.5
MET-Rx® Big-100 Meal Replacement	7.5
Genisoy® Xtreme	7.0
DrSoy Healthy Snacker® Bar	6.5
Genisoy®	6.5
Hershey's SmartZone®	6.5
Think!® Bar	6.5
FIBAR® (all flavors)	6.0
MET-Rx Protein Plus®	6.0
Nutra Blast®	6.0
Promax Carb Conscious®	6.0
Clif® Bar	5.5
Clif Builder's Bar®	5.5
Promax®	5.5
South Beach Diet® Meal Bar	5.5
Slim-Fast Optima® Snack bar	5.0
Ensure®	4.5
SnackWells®	4.5
Nutri-Grain®, Kellogg's® (all flavors)	3.5
GOLEAN® Crunchy, Kashi®	3.0
Melaleuca® Fruit & Fiber Bar	2.5
Melaleuca® Access Activity bar	-1.0
GOLEAN®, Kashi®	-2.0

Most of these snack/health bars are based on some sort of grain or milk product. Those at the top of the list are low in fat and high in fiber and nutrients. Most of the nutrients unfortunately are added in, and are not part of the basic food ingredients. Some are very high in protein rather than carbohydrates. Proteins can be beneficial in keeping blood sugar stable over time whereas the carbohydrates can give a quick source of energy. It is interesting to see that some of the "health" snack bars are not very nutritious at all due to the processing of the ingredients.

Chapter Three on pre- and post-exercise nutrition discusses in detail the use of snack bars in relation to an exercise regime. Any of those with a Nutripoint score of 10.0 or greater would be recommended. In general, however, these foods must be looked at from the aspect of convenience. A runner needing more energy during an event could eat a Power Bar more easily than an orange. But in many cases, the most natural nutrition (nutrients and natural phytochemicals already in the food without being added) would still be convenient for most activities.

The better choices would be some of the following:

High Carbohydrate	Nutripoints
½ c (or 1 whole) Raw Carrots	35.5
¼ Cantaloupe	29.0
6 oz V-8 Juice	28.5
½ Papaya	20.5
1 c Strawberries	19.0
¾ c Currants, Black	19.0
½ Mango	17.5
1 Kiwi	17.0
½ c Mandarin Oranges	15.5
1 Banana	14.0
¼ Honeydew Melon	14.0
2 Plums	14.0
1 Orange	13.5
3 Apricots (or 6 pc dried)	13.5
1 Tangerine	13.0
½ Grapefruit	13.0
½ c Blackberries	13.0
½ c Fruit Salad	13.0
½ c Raspberries	12.5
6 oz Orange Juice	11.5
1 Peach	11.0
6 oz Grapefruit Juice	11.0
1 c Watermelon	10.5

½ c Fruit Cocktail	10.0
1 Nectarine	10.0
Nutripoint Bran Muffin	10.0
Whole Wheat Crackers	9.0
Oat Bran Cereal	7.0

High Protein	Nutripoints
1 c Nonfat Yogurt	10.5
1 c Skim Milk	9.5
½ c Tuna, Canned/water	8.0
Vegetarian Burger	7.5
1 c Lowfat (2%) Milk	7.5
Vegetarian Hot Dog	5.0
½ c Soybean Nuts	5.0
½ c Lowfat Cottage Cheese	4.5
¼ c Sunflower Seeds	4.5
Bean Burrito	4.0
¼ c Healthy Trail Mix	4.0
¼ c Pumpkin/Squash Seeds	2.5
¼ c Unsalted Peanuts	1.5

Note: When totaling your Nutripoint scores for each serving, give more Nutripoints for a larger serving and less Nutripoints for a smaller serving than the standard size. The score given correlates to the standard serving size.

The high carbohydrate snacks are useful for quick energy 10-15 minutes previous to the workout/event or during prolonged exercise sessions. They are also useful immediately following the workout to replenish nutrients, fluids, and immediately increase blood glucose levels.

The high protein snacks are useful 1-2 hours previous to a workout to help maintain sustained glucose levels during the exercise session. See Chapter Three for the complete nutritional program for athlete's pre- and post-exercise.

CHAPTER FIVE

MANAGING STRESS FOR PEAK ENERGY

Peak athletic performance requires peak energy during the competitive event. Physical and mental stress near the time of, or during the event, can decrease or divert energy away from the intended use. Managing stress for the athlete is an important factor in the competitive edge. Some stress is good for competition as it increases the body's readiness for physical activity. The "fight or flight" syndrome explains why the body prepares us in a fearful situation. The readiness for competition psychologically leads the body to physically prepare itself for activity.

The Stress Response

The body's stress response is a normal reaction to a danger signal. The brain perceives a threat and stimulates the hypothalamus, pituitary, and then adrenal glands to pour out catecholamines (speeds heart rate, increases blood pressure, dilates pupils), glucocorticoids (increases blood glucose), and mineralcorticoids (increases blood volume and sodium). All of this enables us to deal with the threat *physically*. During competition, and to some degree training, we are in this "fight or flight" mode.

With the physical activity of training or competition we naturally "burn" these chemicals and hormones secreted by the body, so there can be a balance in training between these chemicals being secreted and burned in a natural cycle. If we all lived in a bubble, this would be controllable and very predictable, but we live in the real world where we have additional psychological stress to deal with. This additional stress can cause us to be in a "chronic" state of readiness to physically act on our fears, thus draining the body of its energy and natural chemical and hormone stores. This can decrease physical performance and cause us to tire more easily during our workouts.

Whether our fears are real or imagined, the body does not know the difference. It gives the same response. Mark Twain once said, "In my time, I have known a great many troubles…but most of them never happened!" Whether real or imagined, a perceived threat or fear will cause the same stress response.

Sources of Stress Today

One stress researcher estimates that today we have approximately 1000 times more stress-producing events in our lifetime than when our great-grandparents lived! The increased technology and pace of society today are making it increasingly more difficult to cope with life. Communication, transportation, information processing, and new knowledge are all making great advances which in some way benefit society. These changes, however, take their toll on us as we are bombarded with more stressful events and less time to recover from each one. Change is the norm. The average American moves 14 times in their lifetime. The average American male will hold 10 jobs in his lifetime.

The Results of Prolonged Stress

Too much stress can result in anxiety, fatigue, depression, insomnia, tremors, and eventually become heart disease, cancer, ulcers, colitis, hypertension, diabetes, and allergies. The immune system is compromised, fats and glucose are dumped into the system, and blood pressure is increased—all causing stress-related diseases—common in today's modern society. For the athlete, it can decrease performance and increase healing time. It can cause you to become injured more easily. It can drain energy so much that you may cut out some training, or be unable to compete altogether.

StressPoints™ to Help You

The athlete can benefit from this 3-point formula designed to help those needing stress-relief and balance in their lives:

1. Try to PREVENT or ELIMINATE THE STRESSOR as your first line of defense.

- Prioritize, and then *don't sweat the small stuff.* Ask: how important is it going to be a year or 5 years from now? Work towards main life goals, don't get bogged down or sidetracked with issues of lesser importance.

- *Spread out life changes* so that you allow time between stress-producing events to recuperate. Any change, whether positive or negative, requires adaptive energy in order to adjust. Plan a buffer time between events if possible to allow for the unexpected.

- *Learn to say "no"* when you really can't handle an additional load. Sometimes pride gets in the way, or we want to be a "nice guy/girl" to others at our own expense. We know better than anyone else what our limits are, so don't let others make you feel guilty.

- *Don't be available and accessible 24 hours a day, 7 days a week.* Take breaks during the day, a day off each week, and vacations during the year. Your body will naturally bounce back if you break up the chronic pattern of the stress.

2. If you can't prevent or eliminate it, MODERATE YOUR PERCEPTION of the stressful event. It could be that the only answer to the problem is a change of attitude.

- *Change your attitude about stressful events you cannot change.* How you *perceive and respond to stress* is determined by *you,* not the event. You decide the price you will pay. React a 1 or 2 instead of 9 or 10. Learn to be "thick-skinned".

- If you are in a no-win situation, try to *pull away from it for a time of relief,* or *change the environment* which causes the situation. Even though the situation doesn't go away, your body will become stronger for the time being.

- Take a look at your stressors and analyze: *"Are my worries based on objective reality or something that has a low probability of occurring?"* Much worry is wasted on things that could occur, but never happen. Be "efficient" in your release of "worry energy".

3. If you can't get rid of the stressor, and it is not appropriate to—or you are unable to change your attitude regarding it, then you can resort to using COPING MECHANISMS to deal with the inevitable stress. These help your body to be as strong as possible to withstand the stress.

- *Get adequate EXERCISE.* Exercise is nature's tranquilizer. It burns up the chemicals and hormones secreted during stress so we can fully relax. Exercise actually puts a *governor effect* on the adrenal glands' response to stress. This is one thing athletes have going for them automatically.

- *Get optimal NUTRITION.* Stress burns up many nutrients including vitamin C and B vitamins. Optimal nutrition helps replenish these nutrients. *Proper nutrition assures the body it is getting all of the nutrients needed to resist disease while under high levels of stress.* Whole foods in their natural form and avoidance of sugar, salt, fat, processed foods, alcohol, and caffeinated beverages can help do this. You can then use Juice Plus+® to make up the difference between your best efforts at eating better, and reaching optimal nutrition.

- *Pure WATER.* Use water inside to cleanse and flush out body wastes, carry out chemical reactions/processes, and provide more endurance. Use it outside to cleanse and relax through saunas and whirlpools/Jacuzzi.

- *RELAXATION.* Use progressive muscle relaxation, massage, heat, sunlight, and biofeedback techniques. Development of the spiritual component of our lives often helps individuals obtain a certain peace and calmness.

- *Express your FEELINGS.* Those who hold things in are at high risk for developing heart disease, hypertension, and cancer. Sharing with a close friend can do wonders for you as you find that you are not alone in your situation—and they can help you make it through similar experiences. Crying can emotionally and physically reduce stress through release of certain chemicals. Strong family, community, church, and group associations correlate highly with ability to handle stress well.

Stress is and will continue to be a part of our lives. Without it, life would be boring and we would have no challenges. We *can*, however, limit unnecessary stress, change our attitudes when we can't change the situations, and strengthen our bodies physically to withstand the inevitable stress we will experience. Using these techniques can help us save the energy we need for training and competition, using it for our best advantage and keeping us healthier in the process.

CHAPTER SIX

THE TRUTH ABOUT POPULAR MYTHS & FADS

THE CELLULITE MYTH

Cellulite is a name for fat deposited under the skin that bulges to produce a dimpled, orange peel appearance, usually on the hips, thighs and buttocks. And though people think it exists, you will not find it in any medical text. In fact, the word cellulite is believed to have been created by some imaginary marketer who realized you have to name a condition before you can promise to cure it.

Advocates of gadgets, gimmicks, and creams to remove cellulite maintain that it is a form of fat gone wrong—a combination of connective tissue, fat, water, and toxic wastes forming a health hazard. Supposedly, the mixture hardens to form characteristic pockets of fat they term cellulite.

Getting Rid of It!

The hope of creams and the so-called "caffeine theory": it will jump start your metabolism, burning off the fat and water thought to cause dimpled skin. The "drill": you rub cream into fatty areas twice daily for at least two months and then only once daily to maintain results. The "claims": skin should be smoother after one month and continue to improve for another five months.

The Reality: the caffeine has a tightening effect that may last a few hours but you can only metabolize fat internally. Though skin may tighten for a few hours, the dimples seen as "cellulite" actually go deep into the fatty tissues. A topically applied product cannot get rid of cellulite.

The Real Scoop

From the view of the scientists, the whole concept of cellulite is irrational; even the term "cellulite" has no scientific meaning. Double blind biopsy studies of fat from people with dimply, lumpy fat tissue and those with normal appearing fat issued clear results: there was no difference in the chemical composition of the fat cells. The difference in appearance of fat is probably caused by an increase in the size of the fat cells. Women tend to deposit more fat in the hips, buttocks and thigh area, which may cause fat compartments to bulge, producing a waffled appearance of the skin.

There is simply no basis in fact that cellulite is different than fat, so don't waste your money on products promoted as cellulite removers. You must lose fat weight before stored fat will decrease. There is no way around it. So called medical treatments like external ultrasound, assisted liposuction, mesotherapy—needles used to inject caffeine into the skin, and Endermologie—intense pressure compressing fat resulting in smoother skin all have been touted as "the answer" and none have been proven to give lasting results. They range in price from $1,000 per treatment and up.

What Really Works

So what do you do? My recommendation is "Burn up the Calories!" resulting in less fat to accumulate. Run, walk, cycle or do any fairly intense exercise three times per week. In fact, one of the truly great exercises for trimming the hips, buttocks and thighs is the Isorobic walk, jog or run. You can go to my website at: **www.JackMedina.com** and clink on "Jack Recommends" to learn more about Isorobic Exercise and see my video demonstration. Or you can call me at 1-866-204-8786.

It is a great exercise program because you are moving against resistance and the body is forced to tilt forward, thus moving the work load back to the buttocks, hamstring and calf muscles. In addition, this program is portable and can be used virtually anywhere. I personally use this program myself and recommend it to everyone.

AMINO ACIDS, PROTEINS AND EXERCISE PERFORMANCE

For years, experts and non-experts have been debating whether or not athletes, particularly those who wish to gain muscle mass, should consume extraordinary amounts of protein in their diets. Protein powders and special amino acid mixtures have held their places among the top sellers in the dietary supplement field.

What contribution does protein make to energy requirements? Does the consumption of carbohydrate speed up the production of protein in muscles? How much protein do athletes in various sports need in their diets? Are proteins good enough, or is it better to consume specific mixtures of amino acids that are purported to improve protein buildup in muscles? Here is what the experts say:

1. **How much of the energy expended during exercise of various types can be attributed to the use of proteins and amino acids as fuels?**

    The majority of energy for all types of exercise is derived from carbohydrates and lipids. For endurance exercise, the estimates vary from 2-3% up to as much as 10 %. There are no estimates for resistance exercise.

2. **What are the basic determinants of whether or not muscle size increases when one trains with resistive exercise?**

    The primary stimuli for determining muscle growth are resistance exercise training and the interaction of the training with food intake. Protein and carbohydrate consumption are secondary to these two considerations.

3. **How much dietary protein should an athlete consume on a daily basis?**

Strength and endurance athletes may need to consume 1.2-1.6 grams of protein per kilogram body weight each day. Still, because athletes typically increase their energy intake during training, they should be able to obtain the protein they need from their ordinary foods and need not resort to special protein supplements. With the possible exception of athletes who are vegetarians, it is extremely unlikely that any athletes in Western countries would need to use protein supplements.

4. **Is it better to consume special mixtures of amino acids to increase muscle growth, or can proteins in ordinary meals do the job just as well?**

Proteins in ordinary meals are probably just as effective as amino acid supplements for increasing muscle growth. In addition, frequent feeding of small meals may be preferable to a single large meal in order to help maintain blood amino acid concentrations over a longer period of time. There is no evidence that consuming special mixtures of amino acids or certain kinds of proteins offers any advantage as far as increasing muscle growth.

5. **How important is it to eat plenty of carbohydrates, in addition to proteins, if one wishes to maximize muscular development?**

To maximize muscular gains, an athlete should be taking in more food energy than is being expended, and carbohydrates should be the major energy source, i.e., at least 50% of the total caloric intake.

6. **Can supplements of branched-chain amino acids (BCAA) taken before and during exercise delay the onset of fatigue?**

The best studies directly testing the effect of consuming BCAA on performance show that BCAA ingestion does not benefit performance. In fact, a potential side effect of BCAA ingestion is an increase in plasma and muscle accumulation of ammonia, which itself can contribute to fatigue. On balance, it appears that ingestion of BCAA is not effective in improving exercise performance. Despite claims to the contrary, branch-chained amino acids do not seem to be important fuel sources during exercise, regardless of intensity, and their is no solid rationale for BCAA supplementation.

Reference: **Sports Science Exchange Roundtable**, Volume 11 (2000)
Kevin Tipton, Ph.D.
Martin J. Bibala, Ph.D
Mark Hargreaves, Ph.D

THE HIGH PROTEIN DIET

A variant on the high-protein/low carbohydrate diet is the "Protein-Sparing Modified Fast during which a person eats only protein. Sound familiar? This regimen is based upon the assumption that protein foods eaten will spare the loss of lean body tissue, and the body will break down its own fat at a maximum rate to meet energy needs. Neither of these assumptions is correct or accurate.

The body's top priority is to meet energy or caloric needs. The normal way to do this is by periodic refueling—EATING! The protein-sparing modified fast provides 450-500 calories in the nine ounces or so of protein usually recommended. The body requires more than double this amount of calories. Thus, all of the protein eaten has to be converted to glucose (a carbohydrate) for the body to meet its energy requirements. The protein eaten is NOT used to replenish the body protein!

If this is true, how does the body meet the caloric deficit remaining after it converts protein foods to glucose? When food is restricted to less than minimum caloric needs the body must find other sources of fuel within its own tissue. After glucose is spent, the body mobilizes stored carbohydrates from the liver and muscles in the form of glycogen. This source however, is exhausted in a matter of hours. At this point most of the body cells are depending on fatty acids (from stored body fat) to continue providing their fuel. However, the brain cells cannot use fatty acids; they need glucose.

Normally the brain consumes up to two thirds of the total glucose used by the body each day. The only other source of glucose left is the body's protein tissue such as muscle, and other parts of the body comprised of protein, which is all expendable. Every cell in your body is composed of some form of protein, which means your body begins eating itself from the inside out. In the first few days on a protein-sparing modified fast (high protein diet), the body protein provides approximately 90% of the needed glucose.

As this regimen continues, the liver is unable to oxidize fat completely. This leads to an accumulation of ketone bodies in the blood and urine. Normally produced and used only in small quantities, ketones can enter some brain cells and serve as their fuel. But ketone production continues to rise until at the end of several weeks is meeting about half or more of the brain's energy needs. Still, about 20% of the brain absolutely refuses to use anything except glucose, and the body protein continues to be sacrificed in order to produce it.

Ketone bodies are acidic and interfere with normal metabolic processes. The risk factors associated with increased ketone bodies, as well as the side effects of this kind of high protein diet are:

Calcium Depletion
Nausea
Dehydration
Kidney Failure or Stones
Weakness
Gout
Arthritis
Arteriosclerosis

Some other effects of this kind of high protein diet include:

- Rapid weight loss within the first 1-2 weeks. This weight loss is due to losses in glycogen, body protein, water and sodium. For each gram of glycogen lost, 3 grams of water are also lost. As the body adapts in 2-3 weeks, water can be retained even to the point of causing weight gain. Weight lost, as water, is regained once normal eating is resumed.

- Contrary to claims being made, this type of diet does not decrease appetite unless it is secondary to other side effects (dehydration, nausea, etc.).

- The safety of this kind of diet has also been questioned. A number of individuals have died of ventricular arrhythmia. The cause of death could not be attributed to the lack of potassium, absence of medical attention, or the protein product used.

The person who wishes to lose body fat will select a balanced diet in the form of complex carbohydrates (fruits, vegetables, grains, legumes and beans; 5-9 servings are recommended daily), protein and fat. At this level body protein will be spared, ketosis need not occur, vital lean tissue will not starve and, body fat will be lost. In combination with an exercise program you will have the tools to lose fat and maintain this loss permanently.

I suggest you check out the websites for the Nutripoints Program (www.Nutripoints.com) and the Isorobic Exercise concept at www.JackMedina.com.

What should I ask before starting this kind of high protein/low carbohydrate diet?

- Ask about the term often used "while under medical supervision"—who is supervising? This diet takes a specialist in this area and eliminates all General Practitioners. Ask his or her qualifications to help you control this program and how often your blood will be analyzed.

- Ask the "Nutritionist" that will be working with you "are you a professional nutritionist or dietician? What qualifies you to advise me on this program?"

- If they are recommending a vitamin/mineral supplement ask them why? Is it because this type of diet is deficient in many of the necessary nutrients and phytonutrients normally found in good food? Research today indicates that vitamin/mineral supplements don't work; they only work if they come in whole food or a whole food supplement.

- Ask, "Can I return to a normal 'American' diet in the future without regaining lost weight?" If the answer is "yes", how can such a blanket claim be made? Where is the research to substantiate this?

Remember, you are interested in losing FAT, not weight. Talk to a real professional in weight management before embarking on a program that can cause major health problems.

HGH – THE LATEST ATHLETIC DREAM DRUG

THE FACTS ABOUT SOMATOTROPIN

Because of the prospect of increased size and reduced fat stores, non-athletes, athletes, and even some parents of young athletes may consider purchasing human growth hormone, also known as Somatotropin. It now competes with anabolic steroids in the illicit market of alleged tissue building, performance-enhancing drugs. HGH is produced in the adenohypophysis of the pituitary gland. Specifically it stimulates bone and cartilage growth, enhances fatty acid oxidation, and reduces glucose and amino acid breakdown.

The U.S. Olympic Committee Drug Education Program has heard from parents who want to help their athletically gifted, but short or average sized children gain additional height. Most of these parents see nothing wrong with such a step, and the children themselves are usually enthusiastic, dreaming of a rich life in professional sports.

At first glance, HGH use may seem appealing to the strength and power athlete. However, few well-controlled studies have examined how HGH supplements affect healthy subjects undergoing exercise training. The use of human cadaver-derived HGH (used until May 1985 by U.S. physicians to treat children of short stature) greatly increases the risk of contracting Creutzfeldt-Jacob disease, an infectious, incurable, fatal brain deteriorating disorder.

Human Growth Hormone is one of the most powerful anabolic substances known to science. It is part of your normal production of hormones every day. Growth hormone output is critical to athletes, since it is a primary stimulus for muscle growth, muscle strength, skeletal growth, tendon growth, injury repair, and mobilization of body fat for energy. This last factor is the reason for its recent resurgence in advertising in magazines, radio and television advertising.

Use by Athletes

Athletes in power sports, such as weightlifting, football and the field events of track and field competitions, are the most likely to experiment with HGH. Most believe it will provide many of the benefits of anabolic-androgenic steroids such as increased muscle mass, but much more safely. Information about its use however, comes mainly from hearsay and brochures distributed through health food stores. Attempts to follow this information are generally a total failure.

Growth hormone is released into the bloodstream by a variety of natural stimuli, including sleep, heat, exercise, food deprivation, hypoglycemia, and certain amino acids and other nutritional manipulations. Any use must be prescribed and precise, and must be based upon science, not hearsay. They cannot be taken orally because growth hormone is destroyed by digestion. In past years, from back alley labs, came "gorilla juice" or "rhesus monkey growth hormone" at up to $800.00 for a three-month supply. It was supposed to be growth hormone extracted from the pituitaries of rhesus monkeys. Only the stupid fall for this one. It is rare, very expensive and has little effect on humans. In fact, the cost alone kept athletes away. It has been calculated that it might cost $10,000 a year to obtain enough to produce an ergogenic effect.

We see athletes who are not even getting what they think is growth hormone. Vials are being falsely labeled. The sellers make big incomes on the black market; they are getting true drug prices for things like saline. Several things are certain at this point: It is 100% certain that growth hormone will be used illegally to promote muscle growth in athletes. It is 100% certain that some athletes will make big gains. It is 100% certain that athletes will use excessive amounts of the drug and will suffer the side effects of acromegaly, including thickening and coarsening of the skin, darkening of the skin, overgrowth of bone ends, hands and feet and skull bones, giving an Ape-man appearance. Especially prominent is the ridge above the eyes and the enlargement of the lower jaw. Additional less visual side effects include insulin resistance leading to type 2 diabetes, water retention, and carpal tunnel compression.

This information, coupled with reports of athletes mega-dosing in the range of 20 times the dosage recommended for therapeutic purposes is frightening. The possible dangers of long-term use of increased endogenous growth hormone levels in healthy people have not been determined. However, HGH is very popular among drug makers. It is highly sought after by manufacturers who want to add it and/or have currently added it to their product line.

Conclusion

Certainly, the legitimate market for growth hormone is good, as it may have some benefit in treating osteoporosis and obesity, although it has not been proven clinically effective for either condition.

Use of growth hormone is a form of cheating, counter to the quest for physical excellence that sport is supposed to honor. The hormone carries risks to health, and ultimately, its use is coercive to other athletes. Parents and coaches would not be fulfilling their function as guardians of their children or athletes' well being by giving them substances that could harm them. At this point the risks far outweigh any advantage which might be gained by taking a chance.

THE TRUTH ABOUT CREATINE

DOES IT WORK?

The American College of Sports Medicine has stated that though some of the research being done shows many gains in strength and muscle bulk for those using creatine, there is NO <u>long-term</u> research that has been done. I have seen many of the short-term studies and must admit they are impressive. However, it is the <u>long-term</u> results I am worried about.

Most supplements are worthless as ergogenic (muscle growth) aids. Most research on supplements shown to help with performance (protein and creatine), have been done on overall lean body mass but not actual changes in the cell itself. It's important to ask whether microscopic changes actually match the changes you see in the mirror. Why? Because this is a narrow-minded attitude. As an example, creatine has been shown to increase water retention, so any gains you see in muscle size may actually be due to more water weight.

Creatine is the most popular supplement available today. Why? Because of all the supplements available, creatine is the only one where the research is quite clear: if you train with creatine, you will probably have bigger gains in strength and body mass than if you trained without it. The type of training and sport that benefit most from creatine are those that require great exertion over a short amount of time, such as all strength and power sports. These range from a 100-meter sprint to a vertical jump and bench press.

However, research on creatine has, for the most part, been done on males. The physiology of a female athlete is significantly different from that of a male. This means that gains a male athlete may experience from creatine may not be true for the female athlete. Most research done to-date has found little or no significant differences between placebo and creatine groups tested after 10 weeks of creatine loading. This means no significant positive effect on strength, strength endurance, or muscle mass in women. There is a lot of difference in testing methodology to determine changes in body mass and strength parameters being measured. These differences, along with other factors such as creatine muscle threshold loading, work load during testing, non-responders, etc. can have significant effects on the research results being published.

There are some serious doubts in the research community about generalizing from a male subject pool to a female subject pool about the effects of creatine. Female athletes should look at creatine supplementation with skepticism until more good scientific research is available.

The human body produces creatine and it is also found in meat products. Research has shown that if you add creatine to your diet, you will probably increase intramuscular levels of creatine, resulting in increased overall training effect. The problem you face is the lack of control over the supplement industry. Manufacturers don't have to tell you exactly what is in the container. There can be things in the container that are not on the label and things on the label that are not in the container. Some manufacturers will do almost anything to make their product better seem better than a competitor's.

The Risks

Creatine is an amino acid produced naturally by the liver and kidneys and stored naturally in muscles. The increased muscle bulk resulting from the use of creatine supplements is largely due to water retention. This is the same as with steroids and human growth hormone which can be extremely dangerous!

The Side Effects that are possible scare me too:

- Hyper-hydration of the muscle, it retains too much water. The heart is a muscle, if it retains too much water, you can die.

- Dehydration of the muscle (some athletes instead of retaining water, lose it). Seventy-eight percent of a muscle is water. If the muscle loses water you immediately begin to lose strength.

- Severe muscle cramping. A professional football player recently ruptured a quadriceps muscle jogging onto the field for the player introductions because of this problem.

- Liver and kidney problems are possible.

How it Works

ATP is the chemical held in the muscle cell which allows the muscle to contract. The creatine, which is GOD-given, allows the muscle to recover the ATP. Therefore, the more creatine in the cell, the faster the recovery after a bout of exercise, therefore more work can be done in a shorter amount of time, therefore quicker strength gains.

Conclusion

How would you feel as a parent if I told your son, "Go ahead and take the creatine, the risk involved is minimal." Then 7 years later he has cancer of the liver because I didn't know! Schools like Michigan State University and UCLA do not allow any supplements of any kind in their athletic programs. This is the kind of school I would want my son to attend.

You can contact the American College of Sports Medicine in Indianapolis, Indiana and request information on their stance regarding creatine. I personally, as a coach and trainer, would NEVER allow an athlete to take a substance where there is no long-term research available. There is already enough creatine in the body to do the job if you are trained correctly. I question the integrity of any person that would recommend this substance to an athlete.

Although creatine, as of this writing, has not been banned by the IOC or NCAA, sooner or later a banned substance will be added to someone's creatine supplement to make it "better." Is it worth the risk? I don't think so.

SCIENTIFICALLY EVALUATING RESEARCH CLAIMS

Whatever happened to professional integrity? The public, with more than 250,000 supplements, combinations of supplements, weight loss products, quick fixes, and instant fitness machines on the market, is being taken advantage of. Professional ethics and integrity have been replaced by "no" ethics and the advertisers desire to get as much out of you, the consumer, as possible. I'm appalled at the infomercials, advertisements, and claims being made that are designed to take advantage of us. Claims that can't be backed up with scientific facts, or "pills" that are supposed to take care of one problem but with "side effects" potentially leading to more problems than you started with.

Even those making the claim "clinical studies" prove that ------, are pulling our legs. What clinical study, where was it done, who controlled the study, was it a well-designed study, where was it published?

Before you buy, ask this question about a "product" before relying on hearsay, claims and testimonials: "Where is the third-party, randomized, double-blind, crossover, peer-reviewed, published research to support what you are saying? Where has this research been duplicated? I want to see it for myself! When you ask this question you eliminate 99% of the "stuff" being touted by advertisers.

There are literally thousands of research studies done every year. It usually takes a minimum of a year to complete a scientific study along with a lot of money invested. Then the statistical analysis has to be done. If the study is worth anything at all, it will be sent to, and evaluated by, a peer review committee (experts in this field) who decide whether or not the study should be published; and only about 50% of all studies reviewed get submitted for publication. Once submitted it is going to take somewhere between 6 months and a year before the study is published; making the study a year old before it is available to read.

Do you think the manufacturers of all the "products" being touted today in magazine, newspapers and television are going to go through this costly and lengthy process before trying to sell it to you? NO; absolutely not.

There are no quick fixes. You can't lay on it, sit on it, shake in it, vibrate in it, get wrapped up in it, rub it on your body or ingest it and get instant results.

This book, though dedicated to a gymnast I had the opportunity coach during summer gymnastics camp many years ago, has been written for those of you (athletes and non-athletes) who are looking for answers based upon "fact", not fantasy.

So the next time you see a TV commercial or read a newspaper or magazine article about a supplement or product and it says "clinical" research says ------, think about the following:

- **Is the research "Third-Party"?** Did the company producing the "product" pay to have another institution or research organization do the research, or was the research done in their own lab or facility with their own people.

- **Was the research "Double-Blind"?** The people taking part in the study have no idea whether or not they are taking a placebo or the real thing. This eliminates any possible "placebo effect", people thinking it made them feel or react differently when in fact it did not.

- **Was the research "Randomized"?** A computer determines who gets what during the study, not the people providing the material (supplement) used. This helps eliminate bias and actual control of results.

- **Was there "Crossover"?** Meaning at some point the placebo group and test groups were reversed to see if results changed accordingly. This is not absolutely necessary for a study to be a good, scientific one, but adds further credibility to the results if it is done, and it confirms the original study.

- Was **"Blood Testing"** for "antioxidant" changes done? Many diseases recently have been associated with "oxidation" in the body, which is a form of "wear and tear". If this test was not done, there is no way to know if a product being tested is effective in an antioxidant capacity.

- Are the results of this study or studies **reproducible**? In other words, could another scientist somewhere else do the same study and get the same results?

- Have the **results of the study been published** in a peer-reviewed "Professional Research" journal? This gives credibility to the study since strict research criteria are usually necessary to get published and peers (who may be skeptical) can evaluate and critique.

- Has the study been **presented at a professional organization** for peer-review? Again, more scrutiny and critique.

Many times a study will not meet all of the criteria above, but the more of them that are met, the "better" the study, meaning the results are more likely to be correct.

Evaluating Research Studies

Some other considerations when evaluating a research study:

Justification - does this particular research represent a "fishing expedition" or does it have sound **scientific rationale** indicating this treatment or supplement should produce an effect?

Are **animals** or **humans** being used in the study? There are significant differences in species, so we can't always make generalizations to humans.

Sex - the interactions between exercise training, and nutritional requirements and supplementation may limit the generalizing of findings to the particular sex being studied.

Age - this often has an effect on the outcome of a study.

Training Status - Fitness and training level can influence the effectiveness or ineffectiveness of a particular diet or supplement. Treatments that benefit the untrained person often have little effect on elite athletes.

Nutrition Baseline - It is clear that a nutritional supplement given to a malnourished group will typically show more improvement in improved nutritional status and exercise performance and response to training.

Health Status - research findings from diseased groups cannot be generalized to healthy populations. An improvement for a group of unhealthy individuals may not carry over to a healthy group.

Conclusions of Studies

Findings should dictate conclusions. Many times investigators take conclusions beyond the scope of the data and make claims that are not supported by the research.

Good statistical analysis must be applied to quantify the results so that pure "chance" did not cause the research outcome. The results must be "statistically significant". The more statistically significant, the more likely (higher the probability) that the results didn't happen by chance and will be shown to be correct over time.

Publicizing Findings of Studies

- **Published in Peer-Reviewed Journal** - It is important to understand that quality research withstands critical review and evaluation by colleagues with expertise in the specific area of investigation. Publication in popular magazines or quasi-professional journals does not undergo the same critical analysis as peer-review. In fact, did you know that self-appointed "experts" in nutrition, sports nutrition and physical fitness pay "big bucks" to eager publishers for magazine space to promote their particular point of view? In some cases the "expert" actually owns the magazine.

- **Findings Reproduced by Other Investigators** - Results from one study do not necessarily establish scientific fact. Conclusions become much stronger and are more easily generalized when support comes from laboratories of independent investigators.

Don't let some ad in the newspaper or infomercial on television affect your good judgment. Make sure the research is there to support the claims being made. As of this writing there are over 61 different "weight loss or fat burning" products being touted in the media; all claiming to be the very best. If this was true how come there are so many saying the same thing? If one of these was supported by good scientific research, peer-reviewed and published it would be front-page news worldwide!

Remember, you can't lay on it, sit on it, shake in it, vibrate in it, get wrapped up in it, rub it on your body or ingest it to get in shape!

Reference: **Sports & Exercise Nutrition** - by William D. McArdle, Frank I. Katch, and Victor Katch.

CHAPTER SEVEN

NEVER, EVER GIVE UP!

Here are some stories of American athletes who, with the odds against them, fought back and "never gave up!"

The Rocky Bleier Story

If you believe in numbers, this guy should have been anything but an NFL Football player. It was January, 1968 and the teams in the National Football League were getting ready to select the athletes they wanted. Rocky Bleier was not at the *head* of anyone's list. In fact, he *wasn't even on* most lists at all.

At that time, 1968, players being considered for NFL teams were given points for their weaknesses and deficiencies. When draft time arrives, a team wants to know how the player they are thinking about taking rates, and their computer pops out a number. The worst rating at that time was 2.5. Above 1.8 and the player was considered not capable of playing professional football. Rocky Bleier ended up with a score of between 2.2 to 2.4, but it gets worse; some scouts said, "I don't think --------can win with this kid on their team." Another said, "I don't think this boy can make any professional club."

There were, however, some intangible things the Pittsburgh Steelers liked about this young man, things they couldn't put in a computer—like "heart." So, when the Steelers, a team that had won only 4 games in 1967, got down to the bottom of their computer list at number 417, Bleier was selected. Rocky was the 417th player selected out of at total of 441 selected in that draft.

Before his rookie year, the army drafted Rocky and sent him to Vietnam. Nine months later, when he returned, his right foot was a half a shoe size smaller than his left; the bottom of that foot had been ripped open by shrapnel along the instep from the heel to the ball, across the big toe and the second toe (which had been splintered); dozens of pieces of shrapnel had pierced his right leg from his foot to his thigh.

As he lay behind clumps of bushes in South Vietnam, wounded, weapon gone, close enough to the enemy to hear them talk, well aware their machine gun could cut through the growth and kill him, wondering if his small, cut-off group would be overrun, he prayed: "Dear Lord, get me out of here if you can. I'm not going to B.S. you. I'd like to say that if you get me out of here alive and okay, I'll dedicate my life to you and become a priest. I can't do that because I know that's not what I'll do. I don't want to promise anything now and then change my mind later when things are going good. I don't want to come to you with a tight-situation prayer if I can't be honest. What I will do is this. I'll give you my life...to do whatever you will...I'm not going to complain if things go wrong. If things are good, I'll share my success with everybody around me. Whatever you want to do, wherever you want to direct me, that's fine. This is the best I can do."

A grenade had exploded at Bleier's feet and the steel plate built into his army combat boots was the only reason he still had a right foot. Muscle and flesh also had been ripped from his left thigh by small-arms fire.

What are you going to do when you get back to civilian life, Rock? "I'm a football player, aren't I?"

Maybe not, when the army lists you as 40-percent disabled. A running back has to start, and push off from a, three-point stance. Push off is a fundamental move for a runner. It allows him to start quickly and change directions sharply.

But calcium deposits that form around broken bones and scar tissue had, in effect, "frozen" the first two toes and adjacent ligament and muscle areas around Bleier's right foot. In addition, muscles on the ball of the right foot had begun to atrophy.

The injuries to the right foot would be Rocky's major obstacle. The other wounds would heal, even though infection had invaded as high as his calf. An operation by army surgeons attempted to cut out the scar tissue and bone spurs in the hopes it, and later in physical therapy, would allow Rocky to regain the flexibility and strength he once had there. The operation was only partially successful, therapy did little, and even electrical stimulation therapy was unsuccessful.

Play Again?

An army surgeon was the first in line to tell him: "Rocky, it's impossible." His old coach, Ara Parseghian at Notre Dame was next, although he couldn't bring himself to tell Rocky directly. He just hoped Rocky would someday be able to walk normally.

When the wounds healed, Bleier began to work out by himself. He thought he would just jog a couple of miles the first day, an easy slow start. At about half a mile, he collapsed, "...crying in deep, convulsive sobs as I gasped for air. My mind was racing with disbelief. After all those years as an athlete—my body skilled, strong, responsive—I was now a physical disaster. My foot hurt, my heart was pounding, I couldn't breathe and I lay there, with NFL training camp three months away. Will I ever play football again?"

Bleier couldn't run. He couldn't walk without extreme pain and was limping badly. But Bleier didn't quit, he devised an inner-sole device that made it possible to run on that right foot without agony and he put himself on a murderous training schedule.

As Rocky's foot began to hurt less, he and his roommate Carl Eller, ran up and down the steps at Kansas State University's football stadium. Rocky reached the point where he could run up and down, bottom to top, full-out, five consecutive times with a 10 pound weight tied to each ankle.

Discharged from the army in July, 1970, Bleier moved in with former Notre Dame teammate Terry Hanratty and Terry's wife Rosemary. Terry took a close look at Rocky and began to worry. "The team's a lot different now than it was in 1968." In fact, new coach Chuck Noll, who had been hired in 1969, was to sweep through the Steeler team that greeted him and only 5 were left by Super Bowl time, 1974. Rocky told his friend "I'd like to give it a shot, and see what happens.

Nine running backs were in camp when he reported and they were competing for 5 spots. The best players make the team. It's not a personality contest, it's a vicious battle for a job and even the wounded Vietnam veteran can expect no special consideration.

Teammates, team Vice-president Art Rooney, Jr., Dr. John Best, the Steelers orthopedic surgeon, the team equipment manager, backfield coach Max Coley and others told Rocky to give it up. Rocky played little during the preseason exhibition games. A week before the season was to start, it was time for the final cut. Coach Noll sent for Rocky and said: "Rock, we put you on final waivers. We think you'll pass through" (not be selected by another club). Rocky argued, "Coach, can't I be sent to the taxi squad or something? I feel good, I can help. I don't want to lose the whole season." What can you say after you've been fired?

"As I began to walk out," Rocky said, "Chuck showed a crack in his impenetrable exterior for the first and only time in my experience. He said, "If you want, you can practice with us today." Rocky suited up, worked out and then left. He was the final man cut.

Then a rare force entered Bleier's life, a 69 year-old man who had owned the team for 39 years and never saw it win even a division title. Bleier received a call the morning after he had been cut. Dan Rooney wanted to see him. Coach Noll had been asked by the vice-president, Art Rooney Jr., if he would mind if Bleier were put on the injured reserve list, thinking that another operation on his right foot would help Rocky. He couldn't play but he would be with the team unofficially and not take up one of the playing spots. Noll agreed.

Surgery was the following day and was successful at removing shrapnel in this foot and scar tissue. Bleier did some scouting jobs for the team as he rehabilitated and began working out on his own. By the eighth week he was back in uniform again, practicing with the team and attending meetings. By the final game of the season, two backs had been hurt and Noll reactivated Rocky so he could get into uniform and sit with the team on the field. Pittsburgh ended the season with five wins and nine losses.

The week before the next training camp Rocky pulled a hamstring muscle in his left leg, just where the bullets had cut out a piece of it. He arrived the first day in camp and ripped the injured hamstring; out of action for 3 weeks. Not being able to play, Rocky was told once again to give it up,

Bleier thought he had three options: 1) wait for the hamstring to heal completely, making it too late in training camp to make the team, 2) continue to practice and pray it wouldn't pull again; and, 3) quit.

Only one made sense to him, strap up the leg and go back to practice. "If I pull it again, I pull it and I'm done. If I don't pull it, maybe I've got a chance." Though he played in a couple of exhibition games and did fairly well, he was once again called into coach Noll's office and was put on waivers (but not claimed by another team).

But Rocky wondered, after trying to persuade him weeks earlier to retire, Noll had kept him. Why? Rocky later found out that backfield coach Max Coley wanted Bleier. In a coaches meeting in 1971, before the season opener, Coley said, "Rocky's the only guy I have who will stick his nose in there and block Dick Butkus."

Bleier played eight games that year, in spite of pulling the injured hamstring again and was on all the special teams. He still wasn't a player of pro caliber, but at least he had accomplished goal number two, he was on the team.

At the first day of training camp in 1972, after spending a great deal of the off season working on increasing his flexibility, he was the fastest back in camp during the 40-yard dashes—unbelievable. Three years of work were beginning to pay off for the tough kid who wasn't supposed to play pro football. When he was whole, he was told to quit and when he was wounded, he wasn't smart enough to listen to anyone. Three years of building strength into his legs and body, the extensive winter, spring and early summer of flexibility exercises—courtesy of Mr. Bleier, Sr. and another intangible: he wanted to be faster.

Rocky's next goal was to show everyone he could play. He did play—every game and the Steelers were 11-3 and a division winner for the first time in their history. Bleier was established—but only on special teams. Rocky wasn't satisfied just playing in every game, he wanted to be a starter.

When he came to the 1973 training camp he was in superb condition; only two men on the team—both offensive linemen—were stronger than Bleier and only two were faster—both wide receivers.

Rocky played on special teams but remained the fifth and last running back in Noll's mind as head coach. The team finished 10-4 and was eliminated by Oakland in the playoffs.

Bleier began the 1974 season beginning to think himself only in terms of special teams. Then came the Players Association strike and Bleier realized that at age 28 he was getting old as far as special teams were concerned. He had been reduced to two specialty teams: kickoff and kick return, logging minimal time as a running back since Franco Harris and Steve Davis started all the exhibition games.

Then against Houston, during the last 5 minutes of the first half, with the offense sputtering, a new running back unit was formed. Noll sent Bleier and Pearson in; Rocky's blocking was superb and Pittsburgh won 13-7.

When Franco Harris came back to the lineup two weeks later, Noll moved Rocky from fullback to halfback and that moved proved to be pivotal for the Steelers and for Rocky. Harris and Bleier jelled and both set career highs in rushing.

It is kind of anti-climactic from here. Bleier's running and blocking were part of a superb machine that won the 1975 and 1976 Super Bowls.

Go back for a moment to the beginning of this story. Recall the point system that was mentioned. Of the starting team in both Super Bowls, no one had rated as poorly as Bleier. His fellow backs, for example, Terry Bradshaw and Franco Harris, were 0.9 and 1.0 respectively.

The world is filled with things built (monuments) to honor this event or that person. Well, Rocky Bleier is a human monument to going after a goal, regardless of the odds and/or setbacks. Out of the debris that was Rocky Bleier in 1970 emerged a running back on a twice world championship football team. And no one except Rocky Bleier anticipated that. Who said God doesn't hear and answer prayers?

The Herb Score Story

Six no-hitters and 3 perfect games in 3 years of high school baseball, a total of 8 hits allowed his entire junior year, brought scouts from 14 of the then 16 major league teams to his family's home. Ten offered bonuses up to $80,000 if he would sign with them (a lot of money at that time); four said, "Tell us your best offer and we'll beat it."

One of the greatest pitchers of all time with the Cleveland Indians, his life changed during his fourth year as a big league starting pitcher. During his fourth start of the season, May 7th, he was pitching in the first inning against the New York Yankees.

He retired Hank Bauer and then up came Gil McDougald, Yankee shortstop. With the count 2 and 2, McDougald swung at a belt-high fastball and lined it back at the pitcher's mound. Score had his eyes turned away in his follow-through and he looked up just in time to see a white flash before the ball hit him squarely in the right eye.

Herb never lost consciousness and asked only one question of the hospital physician: "Am I blind?" His physician made him lay still for 8 days until the swelling subsided enough around the eye so Dr. Charles Thomas could clearly evaluate the damage. The retina had been torn, but not completely, and Score would not be blind but might have a blind spot. His vision was blurred for almost a year and no one knew if he would ever pitch again. Herb couldn't tell if a ball thrown to him was 3 or 30 feet away. Exercises during the winter brought his depth perception back and he reported to spring training saying, "I've got to know if I'm gun shy and now is as good a time as any."

If this wasn't bad enough, he injured his arm on his return to the starting lineup, tearing a tendon—but tried to pitch anyway—literally "aiming" the ball rather than throwing it. He was ultimately sent down to the minors hoping he might be able to pitch again. In 1962 and 1963, he attempted a comeback with the Indianapolis where he had started his career. "I didn't want to think 15 years later that I could have pitched if I had tried a little longer. I went out and proved I couldn't pitch." Then it was time to stop.

As a measure of the respect men throughout baseball had for him, he was immediately asked to come back to Cleveland to broadcast its games. Score had created a legend quite apart from his baseball playing: a good man with the potential for athletic greatness who didn't complain when the vision died young.

Courage belongs to people like Herb Score who labor, after injury, with little success for 6 years hoping they may find some part of their former brilliance. He could have quit many times, and I know of many who have quit for less.

On the morning that Herb and his wife Nancy's second child was born, Herb was scheduled to speak before a father and son Communion breakfast at their church. Nancy insisted he go even though he didn't want to. Herb spoke without notes and without mentioning what had happened that morning—no one there knew until later. He spoke of family, of love, of doing one's best at whatever one does and of accepting what life offers without complaint. He could have been thinking of his "damaged" daughter; he could have been thinking of a throwing arm that mysteriously died. Those who were there said no talk of Herb's ever moved them more.

The Y.A. Tittle Story

Y.A Tittle had been the starting quarterback for the San Francisco 49ers for 13 years. Suddenly he was benched in favor of a new quarterback named John Brodie.

At times Y.A. thought, "The hell with it. Quit the damned game. You've been at it too long anyway, and you've got an insurance business that can support your family."

"But the next instant, I'd get stubborn: Come back for another season and show them you're still a good quarterback." Y.A. had been part of the 49ers all these years and now was no longer wanted. Traded to the New York Giants for a rookie lineman, he decided to quit, but was talked out of it by Frank Gifford, his best friend.
Y.A.'s coming to New York took courage!

During Tittle's first play of the exhibition season against the Los Angeles Rams he bobbled the handoff and fell on the ball. A half ton of Rams fell on him—and cracked several bones in his back. Out for five weeks.

Yet the 1961 season and the eastern division title "was just like being born again." In August, after coming to New York, Tittle had no one to even have dinner with. Four months later, the Giants gathered in a New York restaurant to celebrate winning the eastern division championship and when all the speeches and tributes were done, a spontaneous clamor went up around the room: "Y.A, Y.A., Y.A.," and the same bald man slowly rose and talked about the "greatest year in my life."

In 1962 the Giants won 12 of 14 games and Tittle tied a league record by throwing seven touchdown passes in one game against Washington. In 1963, at age 36, Tittle led the Giants to a division title for the third consecutive year.

After retiring at age 38, Y.A. came back to the Giants as quarterback coach. He is a legend in the Pro Football Hall of Fame. He never, ever, gave up!

WHAT IT TAKES TO BE NUMBER ONE

The following is a speech given by the great Vince Lombardi. It is entitled, "What it Takes to be Number One". I have this article framed above my desk and I see it every day and it motivates me to do my very best every day.

"Winning isn't a sometime thing, it's an all the time thing. You don't win once in awhile, you don't do things right once in awhile; you do them right all the time.

There is no room for second place. There is only one place in my game, and that's first place. I have finished twice in my time at Green Bay and I don't want to finish second again. There is a second place bowl game, but it is a game for losers, played by losers. It is, and always has been an American zeal to be first in anything we do, and to win, and to win, and to win.

Every time a football player goes to ply his trade he's got to play from the ground up—from the soles of his feet right up to his head. Every inch of him has to play.

Some guys play with their heads. That's OK. You've got to be smart to be number one in any business. But more importantly, you've got to play with your heart, with every fiber of your body. If you're lucky enough to find a guy with a head and a lot of heart, he's never going to come off the field second.

Running a football team is no different than running any other kind of organization—an army, a political party or a business. The principles are the same. The object is to win—to beat the other guy. Maybe that sounds hard or cruel. I don't think it is.

It is a reality of life that men are competitive and the most competitive games draw the most competitive men. That's why they are there—to compete. They know the rules and objectives when they get in the game. The object is to win the game fairly, squarely, by the rules—but to win.

And in truth, I've never known a man worth his salt, who in the long run, deep down in his heart, didn't appreciate the grind, the discipline. There is something in good men that really yearns for discipline and the harsh reality of head to head combat.

I don't say these things because I believe in the "brute" nature of man or that men must be brutalized to be combative. I believe in God and I believe in human decency. But I firmly believe any man's finest hour—his greatest fulfillment to all he holds dear—is the moment when he has to work his heart out in a good cause, and he's exhausted on the field of battle—victorious."

CHAPTER EIGHT

GROWING STRONGER THROUGH PERSONAL CHALLENGES

How you respond to the challenge of "Training and Fueling your body for Peak Performance" is entirely up to you! In this last chapter I will share some examples of what other people have done when faced with enormous challenges.

Picture this in your mind. A track race, a guy or girl coming off the curve, lungs burning, tired, and about 120 yards to go. Whether this person picks up those knees and drives on or whether they let down and slacken the pace tells you something about this person's will; what they will do in any circumstance in living—how they will respond to a challenge.

A great historian once said, "You can measure a people by the way they respond to a great moment of challenge." This is what life is, a great challenge or cataclysmic moment, and the response that people make to that challenge.

We live in a challenging era today and I can't list all of the challenges here, but these are the basic ones I think we are being confronted with today:

The challenge of using man's genius for that which creates, rather than that which destroys.

Albert Einstein, one of the greatest scientists in history said this: "Our problem is not more science; our problem is directing the genius of man in using what he knows in that which benefits humanity rather than in destroying humanity." We don't want for genius in this country, there is unbelievable talent here. The challenge is to get it going in the right direction.

The challenge of health.

This hit home when I was at the University of Columbia in New York City speaking at a Strength & Conditioning Coaches Conference. We were being held up in traffic, waiting patiently, as a college student was waiting for his buddy. The buddy came out of the building he was in, sauntered down the walkway and got into the car; I'm not exaggerating here, the car drove exactly a half a block around the corner, stopped and the guy got out and went on to his next class. I couldn't help thinking how this illustrates the problems of our time. We have unbelievable machines and mechanization, but we are losing our physical vitality. I maintain that there is a relationship between the physical discipline of the body and what a nation is mentally and spiritually. If we are getting soft physically it's a good indication that something is happening to us mentally and spiritually as well. Here is another great challenge: in an age of softness and complacency to be a dynamic, energetic person physically.

The challenge of brotherhood in an age of crisis; this age-old problem of learning to live together as human beings.

I assert to you that unless we can learn to live together as people, one common humanity under one common God, that there won't be any humanity at all unless this happens. All men are created equal; God endows all men with the right of life, liberty and the pursuit of happiness. This American dream can help solve one of the basic problems of the world. It's an enormous challenge and each and every one of us can take a part in making this become a vital part of our lives; breaking down prejudice and asserting brotherhood. It's one of the great challenges confronting democracy today.

You and I know that the real crux of the matter is not the challenge itself but rather the response we make to that challenge. Your action and my action. It's one thing to be theoretical; it's another to put the conviction of your life into your action. Of course, it's easy to respond negatively isn't it? Easy for a person to say what can I do, I'm only one lone guy in a vast world, what can I do?

I think of a guy walking the streets of Vienna, Austria; a wood-be artist, but half crazed with these ideas of racial supremacy. I think of this guy riding social opinions into power, riding the crest of political favoritism to become the Chancellor of Germany and of the Third Reich. Sixty million men and women lost their lives because of the half-mad ideas of that one lone man.

On the creative side, I think of a guy born in a lean-to, Abraham Lincoln, a man without formal education but a man, when the nation was being split apart, held it together in union and became the greatest president this nation has ever known. Individuals do change cultures. Don't say there is nothing you can do; and don't respond by dodging the issues. Any of you who have ever played football know this, there comes a time when that guard or that tackle have got to meet the opposing lineman and they have to square off on the guy. Now they can slide off of him, they can bury their head in the dirt and say, "I tried", but there comes a time when if the team is going to function, that lineman has got to square off, hit the guy and move him out of there. That's the way a team goes. Don't dodge the issues and don't give up. This is why I love the sports world because the sports world lives with challenges, and the sports world lives with responses. You cannot just theorize. You've got to make a decision and act upon it—right now!

A Runner's Challenge and Growth

I think of the story of Herb Elliott from Australia, a great would-be runner, who hurt his foot when he dropped a piece of furniture on it, and more or less drifted into indifference on it. One day he was watching the Olympic Games in Melbourne, Australia and watched John Landy coming around the curve and got a dream. He said to his father "I want to run a mile in under four minutes."

He went up to one of the great Australian coaches and said "I want to be a great runner; I want to run a mile in under four minutes." The coach looked at this 19 year old boy and said "Do you know what it is to run a mile in under four minutes? Do you know what it's like to run when you can hardly feel your legs, when your lungs are burning with fire, do you know what this is?" Herb Elliott said "Sir, I don't care what it takes; I want to run a mile in under four minutes." The coach said, "Okay come on down to the track".

But he didn't put him on the track; he took him on down to the beach and made Herb Elliott run in the sand. He made him run in the sand dunes until he could hardly stand, he made him lift weights until his arms could hardly function, he made him swim until he could hardly take a stroke; he made that boy hurt so bad, then asked him "How do you feel?" Herb said, "I'm still going to do it." The next day he came back again and the coach gave it to him even harder, made him train harder than the day before. To make the story short, six months later Herb Elliott ran the mile in 3:59.4. One month after that he ran it in 3:54.6. In Rome in the 1960 Olympic Games Herb Elliott, as a 21-year-old boy, ran the mile in the equivalent of a 3:51.00.

Do you see what I mean by an immediate response? In six months Herb Elliott had accomplished his dream. It is unbelievable and yet this is what happens in the sports world.

A High School Athlete's Challenge and Growth

Bob Richards, Former Olympic Gold Medalist, tells this wonderful story. He was in Kingsburg, California to give a speech to the high school student body. Later that day he was working out with this big 6'3" kid, running the hurdles, throwing the shot put-discus, and pole vaulting. After the workout Bob said to this kid, the Student Body President of Kingsburg High School, "Say young man, you ought to be a Decathlon Man, you've got a lot of ability." This young boy looked Bob Richards in the eye and said, "Sir, that's what I want to be, I want to be a great Decathlon Man." Six months later, that high school senior beat Bob Richards in the Pan American Games. One month after that he broke Bob Mathias' world record that the experts had said would never be broken; Rafaer Johnson broke it in seven months of intensive training and dreaming. Do you get my point? Men and women, if there is one thing you must learn it's this: If you you're going to do something, BEGIN NOW! You show me a boy or girl who will study for six months and I'll show you a transformed intellect. The thing is we just don't get around to it. The crisis of our hour calls for an immediate response, so respond now.

Faith—the Greatest Power

Faith is the greatest power in the world! Not only faith in yourself, but faith in other people. Carl Erskine, the former great pitcher for the Dodgers tells this story: He was pitching in the World Series, he was ahead and his team was leading the series three games to two. He walked a man, didn't think too much about it, and walked another man. Then big old Johnny Mize came to the plate and as Carl put it, "I slipped a pitch into just the wrong place." Johnny Mize lifted it into the cheap seats of Brooklyn Stadium for a home run.

Now the score was 5 to 5 and all of a sudden the whole complexion of the series had changed. Carl said, "I died on that mound, something inside me just quit. I was worthless. To know that I had let my teammates down like that!" Charlie Dressen, who was then coaching the Dodgers, came off the bench and walked up to Carl, put his hand on his shoulder and said, "How do you feel?" Carl said, "I lied," and said, "I feel pretty good." Dressen could see it, he gripped Carl's shoulder tightly and said, "You're my man Carl, you can do it!" turned abruptly and walked off.

Erskine, when telling this story said, "You can't know what that guy did for me in that moment. To know that he believed in me; that when I failed, that guy was with me." Erskine retired the next 16 men that faced him in the series. Two days later he set a World Series strikeout record.

What do you think would happen if parents would have more faith in their children? What if instead of sermons and lectures there was this something, "I Believe in YOU!" Faith can change everything. The Bible says, "Only believe, all things are possible if you will only believe."

Courage and Fighting Heart

This is a hard one, but if you've ever been in the sports world you know what courage is. When a person stays in there and battles against the odds. Not just as it applies to sports is the quality illustrated by Babe Zaharias, possibly the greatest female athlete of all time, if not the greatest athlete of all time. All-American Softball, All-American Basketball, 3 Gold Medals in the Olympics, one of the greatest women golfers who ever lived, then in the height of her career—cancer. Her husband, George, told how this girl, in the middle of this tragedy, the last day or so before she died, reached out and held his hand saying, "Don't take on so honey, since I've been in this hospital I've learned one thing: a moment of happiness is a lifetime—and I've had a lot of them." This in my mind is <u>courage</u> in human life.

You see it personified in a guy named Harold Connolly, former

World Record holder in the Hammer Throw, waving a big right arm at 100,000 people in a moment of glory. If you could have seen that guy's right arm you would have thought, "No wonder he's the world champion." His biceps muscle is 18" around. But the thing you don't see under the blue USA uniform is a crippled left arm, one-third the size of his right, 4 inches shorter. When he was a kid, because of a freak bone disease, he broke that arm 13 times and it never healed properly.

But this guy does push-ups with this arm, lifts weights with this arm; he does chin-ups with that left arm working. On his third throw in Melbourne, Australia he stepped into the ring with two Russians way out in front of him beyond the World Record. Here is what I'm getting to—the heart of it! As this guy with a crippled left arm unknown to the crowd, puts that crippled left hand on the handle of the hammer, the right hand on top of it, breathes a prayer that GOD will help him do his best; then with that 16 pound ball whirling around his head at a terrific centrifugal speed, leans back at a forty-five degree angle, turns his body 3 times as fast as he can, plants his feet and lets go with a big grunt. And you hear it! A hundred thousand people sucking in air at the same time as the ball hangs in the air, turning-turning and then ker-splat as it hits the ground with the roar of the crowd. You look over at this guy, as he doesn't believe it at first, then a smile breaks out on his face and he lifts that big old right arm in triumph!

You get at life with a story like this because what that boy did with that crippled left arm is what people can do in living. What he did in odds like that to become the World Hammer Throw Champion is what people can do in any realm of life if they have the spirit.

The Spirit

This "spirit" shows up in a young girl named Shelly Mann, a former Olympic Champion swimmer. She was asked during an interview, "How did you get into swimming?" and she told this story. When she was 5 years old she had such a severe case of polio that she could hardly move a muscle. She got into a swimming pool not to become World Champion, but to just put a little strength into those feeble arms and legs. The story of a girl, who at first was held up in the buoyancy of the water; who's goal was to swim 30 feet, just the width of the pool. She struggled through the months of numbness and pain until she could finally make it to the other side of the pool. Then she wants to swim a length, then 2 lengths. She at one time held 8 American records. Then you watch her during the award ceremonies at the Olympics, tears in her eyes, half-crying, half-laughing, clutching in her hand a Gold Medal that at one time she couldn't even hold up. This girl has "fighting heart!" Battling against the odds!

What greater story than the Hungarian who looks down the gun barrel at the bulls-eye, splits it again and again, wins the Gold Medal with his right hand. Then 6 months later loses it in a freak accident. Believe it or not, three and a half years after this tragedy the same guy comes back to Melbourne, Australia, looks down the barrel of the gun at the bulls-eye, splits it again and again, winning his second Gold Medal with his left hand.

In stories like this you see the depths of human life. Remember this: Life does not determine a champion, a champion always determines life. These are stories about what people can do if they have that kind of spirit and kids can see it, not in abstract terms, but they can see it in their hero's, in their ideals.

I think of Charlie Boswell, eyes ripped out of his head in World War II serving his country. I think of this guy who was an All-American halfback, 205 pounds of muscle meeting life's greatest challenge. This guy takes up golf, swinging at a ball he can't even see, putting by sound as someone rattles a metal object in the hole. This guy shoots 36 for 9 holes totally blind. That's par, in case you're interested.

I don't know how many of you play golf, I happen to love the game and I can see everything there is on that whole course, my vision is wonderful. And that's exactly where I am when I play golf, all over the whole course. And I think of a guy without eyes, in a game requiring depth perception and judgment, shooting par! You know what Charlie Boswell said? "Nothing can beat you if you've got a fighting heart!"

My personal mentor and friend Dr. Don Swartz, DC, PT, whom I refer to in an earlier chapter, was blinded in an automobile accident when he was 16 years old. He completed Chiropractic College and Physical Therapy School "blind." Dr Swartz was one of the best, if not the very best, in the world. His personal resume would blow your mind. I owe my knowledge and success as a trainer to this wonderful man who battled the odds after this tragic accident. Don helped and inspired people for over 60 years in Hayward, California.

Forgive another personal reference here, but when I was born my mother was told I would never walk because I didn't have enough blood circulation from the hips down. She refused to believe the medical people. She massaged my legs every day for hours until, against all odds, at age 3 I took my first step. Then they said I would never run, and I ran. People said I would never make it through college. I refused to believe I couldn't do it, receiving my Masters Degree in Physical Education from San Jose State College in 1965 and achieving my goal to become a teacher and coach.

The sports world taught me and can teach kids one of life's greatest secrets: Battle ON! Don't give up! In spite of handicaps, hurt, and setbacks—battle on! There is no better lesson in life.

PERFECTION

I think of striving for perfection. You have to be around the great athletes of the world to appreciate this. Strange as it may seem, for most of them, no matter how good they are, they think they can be better. That's why they are champions. If they have a flaw they work on it hundreds of hours to eliminate it.

A great example here is Bobby Morrow, former Sullivan Award Winner as a sprinter in track and field. I wish you could see this kid work on his "starts." Bobby worked for two hours one day on nothing but the first 25 yards of his race. When he would come up to the start "get set" position he wouldn't move a muscle, he would be just waiting for the starter's gun to go off. It was odd in contrast to the other guys because they were trying to beat the gun. They would be lunging out, coming back, twitching; or they would do it slightly by leaning forward, then lean a little bit more. Bobby wouldn't even attempt that. Bobby's coach said, "He has never tried to beat the gun in his whole competitive career. He thinks it is unsportsmanlike, un-Christian, to get a jump on a competitor." Do you believe this? He single handedly taught a great lesson. He demonstrated that he was better off.

Bobby Morrow said to his coach, "Watch me from behind, if there is the slightest quiver, tell me." His coach would say, "There was a slight tremor on your third step." Bobby would work on it until the tremor was gone. He measured his steps to the quarter of an inch, trying to get the spike marks in the same place. Sports Illustrated magazine described this great Gold Medal winner so beautifully: "Bobby Morrow is 41 Seconds of Blazing Perfection." What a great description of perfection in action.

You have to watch Pat McCormick, one of the best divers of all time. I don't know how many of you have ever watched power-diving. Thirty-five feet up, they go off this platform going 35 miles per hour as they hit the water like a bullet.

Bob Richards tells a wonderful story about watching divers, including Pat McCormick, go off this tower and thought to himself, "That looks so easy, I mean it's only twice 15 feet or so, I ought to be able to do that." So Bob got his swimsuit on and made his way up the ladder to the top of the diving tower. He said, "Have any of you ever gone up a 35 foot tower?" He said, "I got up there and was waving at all of my buddies who were down on the pool deck just waiting for the kill, and I made my first mistake right in the beginning, I looked down! When you do it, don't look down! I just froze!"

"Finally, I looked over the edge and I found the pool and I

would have gone right back down the ladder but for the fact there were a bunch of girls down on the pool deck and I had to prove my masculinity. Well, I took one gulp of air and went off the tower. You know, I was wrong, the first 5 feet is wonderful. You can see everything there is to see, but watch out for that last 30 feet. It's kind of a whistling noise going past your ears, kind of a 'Swoosh' and you think you're almost there and you still have 20 feet to go. From there on it's prayer all the way in. All of sudden "BLAM" I hit the water, my arms collapsed, my head almost flew off. Believe me, you haven't lived until you have gone off just once."

Bob came out of the pool so glad he had all of his body parts and his appreciation grew by leaps and bounds for those kids who do this, especially this girl Pat McCormick. Pat would go off the tower 25-30 times, every dive seeming to be poetry in motion. She would split the water without as much as a ripple and her coach, who happened to be her husband, would say, "Your form wasn't quite perfect, your toes weren't pointed, there was an imperfection here and here." Nobody else could see it! So Pat would set her jaw and go back up the tower repeating the dives for 3-4 hours working on pointing her toes.

Bob Richards said, "I was so happy to still have all ten left after going off the tower, and here is this girl worried about pointing the confounded things." You watch her as she works and works, then in the Diving Finals wins two Gold Medals in Helsinki just 6 months after giving birth to a baby boy. Then 4 years later wins those same two Gold Medals, unprecedented in Olympic competition. The Sullivan Award winner, Outstanding Woman Athlete in the World. Why? Pat says, "With every dive I strive to be better."

You can't be content with mediocrity, you can't have flaws. Watch gymnasts, whom I have been watching for the past 38 years, lose by a 100th of a point. Well in the sports world you've got to keep working. A flaw can ruin a product, men can become drunks with one drink, and one misstep can ruin a young man or woman's character. Life is very much like sports. I suggest you try to adopt this philosophy:

Go up an inch at a time. With every dive, every at bat, every routine, every shot, strive to be better. What a great philosophy for living.

Respond NOW!

You and I know the enormous problems we face. But if ever the world needed men and women who would use their creative genius for that which builds, it's now. If ever the world needed healthy, strong, dynamic men and women, it's now. If ever the world needed brotherhood, personal concern; if ever the world needed answers to its economic problems, if ever the world needed a spiritual perspective in an age of materialism it's now. Men and women, don't respond in fear, don't say there is nothing I can do, don't give up. Don't dodge issues or evade the questions. Right now with a sense of the power and purpose of GOD, with faith and courage, go out and do something about the world. It can be changed!

I think of eleven men who responded to the greatest challenge the world has ever known; two simple little words, "Follow Me." Eleven men, the might of the Roman Empire against them, without wealth, without much education, without much power, but with faith and courage and a sense that the universe was behind them, responded immediately, changed the world.

So can you and I.

SOME FINAL THOUGHTS

From: Jack Medina

It has been 45 years now (though it doesn't seem like it) between my first teaching/coaching job at Homestead High School in Cupertino, California (1962) and the publication of the 2nd Edition of this book. I have always thought about trying to put together the things I have learned during that time, and thought could help others, into print.

Many people have contributed to what you have just read. I attended a seminar many years ago given by Dr. Scott Connelly, M.D. who at that time was at University of Stanford Medical Center. I was intrigued by how simple and interesting he made the complicated subject of Nutrition. I took notes like crazy and I thank him for creating my first real interest in nutrition fact and fantasy. The things he taught me then are still true today.

I met Dr. Barry Brown, Ph.D. who teaches Exercise Physiology at the University of Arkansas who quickly changed my thinking on how the body uses its energy systems and how to apply this information to training athletes. And then I had the good fortune to meet Dr. Roy Vartabedian, author of "Nutripoints" sometime after his book was introduced and became an International Bestseller. We quickly became close friends and business associates.

Roy encouraged me to share my knowledge on working with athletes with others and together we have joined forces to bring you this second edition of *"The Winning Edge: Fueling & Training the Body for Peak Performance"*. With the support and encouragement from my lovely wife Kathy, and my kids Randy, Marjorie and Kelly I was able to spend the hours necessary to put my thoughts in writing. I sincerely hope you have found this material worthwhile and will share it with others. Thanks!

Jack A. Medina, M.A.—President, Designs for Fitness

From: Dr. Roy Vartabedian

Once you meet Jack Medina, you will never be the same. I had the privilege of meeting him almost 15 years ago, and we became instant friends and close business partners. Jack has taught me a lot (and made me laugh a lot!). I knew he had some interesting information from his learning and experience, and wanted him to put his thoughts and knowledge in the field of Exercise and Nutrition in printed form so others could benefit. It's been a pleasure, as always, working with him on this project.

To this I have added my contribution based on the Nutripoints and Stresspoints Programs. My wife, Renée, has contributed with her section on the benefits of Chiropractic to the athlete and active person. We plan to keep it a work in progress, and make updates when necessary to keep up with current knowledge.

We wish you all the best for a happy, healthy future!

Roy E. Vartabedian, Dr.P.H., M.P.H.—President, Designs for Wellness

REFERENCES AND RESOURCES

Coach's Guide to Nutrition and Weight Control – by Patricia A. Eisenman, Stephen C. Johnson and Joan E. Benson, Second Edition, 1990. Leisure Press, a division of Human Kinetics Publishers, Inc., Box 5076, Champaign, IL 61825.

Coach's Guide to Sports Injuries – by J. David Bergeron and Holly Wilson Greene, 1999. Human Kinetics Publishers, Inc. Box 5076, Champaign, IL 61825.

Designing Resistance Training Programs – Steven J. Fleck and William Kraemer, Third Edition, 2004. Human Kinetics Books, Champaign, IL.

Eat Smart, Play Hard – by Liz Applegate, Ph.D. - Rodale Press. 2001.

Exercise Physiology - Energy, Nutrition, and Human Performance – by William D. McArdle, Frank Katch and Victor Katch - Sixth Edition, 2007; Lea & Febiger, Philadelphia/London.

Fitness & Health – by Brian J. Sharkey, Ph.D., Fifth Edition, Human Kinetics Books, Champaign, IL, 2002.

Getting Stronger – by Bill Pearl and Gary T. Moran, Ph.D., Shelter Publications Inc., 1986, by Bill Pearl and Shelter Publications, Inc., P.O. Box 279, Bolinas, CA. 94924.

Gifford on Courage – by Frank Gifford with Charles Mangel, 1976. M. Evans and Co., Inc., New York, N.Y., 10017.

Gold Medal Nutrition – by Glenn Cardwel, ADP, Fourth Edition, Human Kinetics Books, Champaign, IL, 2006.

High Performance Nutrition – by Susan M. Kleiner, Ph.D., R.D., John Wiley & Sons, Inc., 1996.

Journal of Pure Power – by Dan Wagman, Ph.D., CSCS, online journal at www.jopp.us, 2007.

Maximize Your Training: Insights from Leading Strength and Fitness Professionals – edited by Matt Brzycki, Coordinator of Health Fitness, Strength and Conditioning Programs, Princeton University. Masters Press, NTC/ Contemporary Publishing Group, 2000.

Muscle – Confessions of an Unlikely Body Builder – by Samuel Wilson Fussell, Poseidon Press, 1994.

Nancy Clark's Sports Nutrition Guidebook – by Nancy Clark, M.S., R.D., Second Edition,1997. SportsMedicine Brookline, Brookline, MA.

Physical Golf: The Golfer's Guide to Peak Conditioning and Performance – by Neil Wolkodoff, Kickpoint Press, Greenwood Village, Colorado, 1997.

Physiology of Fitness – by Brian J. Sharkey, Ph.D., Third Edition, Human Kinetics Books, Champaign, Illinois, 1990.

Physiology of Sport and Exercise – by Jack H. Wilmore, Ph.D. and David Costill, Ph.D., Third Edition, Human Kinetics Books, Champaign, IL, 2004.

Sport Physiology for Coaches – by Brian J. Sharkey, Ph.D. and David E. Gaskill, Ph.D., Human Kinetics Books, Champaign, IL, 2006.

Sports & Exercise Nutrition – by William D. McArdle, Frank I. Katch, Victor L. Katch, Second Edition. Lippincott Williams & Wilkins, 2005.

Sports Physiology – Second Edition, Edward L. Fox, Saunders College Publishing, 1984.

Sports Supplements – by Jose Antonio, Ph.D., CSCS and Jeffrey R. Stout, Ph.D., CSCS. Lippincott, Williams & Wilkins, 2001.

The Vegetarian Sports Nutrition Guide - by Lisa Dorfman, M.S., R.D., L.M.H.C. John Wiley & Sons, 2000.

The Charlie Francis Training System – by Charlie Francis and Paul Patterson, TBLI Publications, 1992. Printed in Canada.

Total Training for Young Champions - by Tudor O. Bompa, Ph.D., York University, 2000. Human Kinetics Publishers, Inc., Box 5075, Champaign, IL 61825.

INDEX

ORDER FORM

Name:

Address:

Phone: E-mail Address:

	Quantity	Price	Total
The Winning Edge: Fueling & Training			
the Body for Peak Performance	_____	$29.95	_____
Shipping/Handling	_____	5.95	_____
Nutripoints Complete Program			
(Book, QuickStart Audio, Wallchart,			
Daily Record Sheet & Pen, Personal Ed. Software)	_____	$119.00	_____
Shipping/Handling	_____	11.95	_____
Software for Tracking Nutripoints			
Personal Edition (1-user)	_____	$79.00	_____
Family Edition (up to 5-users)	_____	119.00	_____
Professional Edition (unlimited # of users)	_____	249.00	_____
Shipping/Handling	_____	5.95	_____

Isorobic Exercise System (Call 1-866-204-8787 for special pricing)

Subtotal			_____
Sales Tax (for CA deliveries)		7.75%	_____
		TOTAL	_____

Prices valid through December 31, 2007

Send order form along with check, money order, or credit card info to:

Vartabedian & Associates	or	Phone: 1-888-796-5229
P.O. Box 1671		Fax: (760) 804-5996
Carlsbad, CA 92018-1671		**www.Nutripoints.com**
		www.JackMedina.com

***Optionally order online at* www.Nutripoints.com/order.html

Card #:

Circle Card Type: MC   VISA   AMEX

Signature: